Reshaping
Herbal
Medicine

For Churchill Livingstone

Publishing Manager: **Karen Morley**
Development Editor: **Kerry McGechie**
Project Manager: **Caroline Horton**
Design Direction: **Andy Chapman**

RESHAPING HERBAL MEDICINE

Knowledge, Education and Professional Culture

Edited by

Catherine O'Sullivan
Chair of European Herbal Practitioners Association
Education Committee and formerly Vice-Principal,
Newman College of Higher Education, Birmingham, UK

Foreword by HRH The Prince of Wales

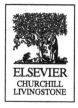

ELSEVIER
CHURCHILL
LIVINGSTONE

ELSEVIER
CHURCHILL
LIVINGSTONE

An imprint of Elsevier Limited

First published 2005

ISBN 0 443 10135 3

British Library Cataloguing in Publication Data
A catalogue record for this book is available from the British Library

Library of Congress Cataloging in Publication Data
A catalogue record for this book is available from the Library of Congress

Note
Knowledge and best practice in this field are constantly changing. As
new research and experience broaden our knowledge, changes in practice,
treatment and drug therapy may become necessary or appropriate. Readers are
advised to check the most current information provided (i) on procedures
featured or (ii) by the manufacturer of each product to be administered,
to verify the recommended dose or formula, the method and duration of
administration, and contraindications. It is the responsibility of the practitioner,
relying on their own experience and knowledge of the patient, to make
diagnoses, to determine dosages and the best treatment for each individual
patient, and to take all appropriate safety precautions.
To the fullest extent of the law, neither the publisher nor the editor
assumes any liability for any injury and/or damage.

The Publisher

Transferred to Digital Print 2007

Printed and bound by CPI Antony Rowe, Eastbourne

Contents

Section One: Knowledge, education and professional culture

Section Two: The traditions of herbal medicine

Section Three: Problems with knowledge, education and culture in the development of the herbal medicine profession

For my parents, Jack and Marianne Watt

Contributors

Peter Conway

Peter is a practising medical herbalist, teacher and author. He came to study herbal medicine following a growing interest in green issues and alternative health approaches. He graduated from the 4-year full-time course in herbal medicine at the College of Phytotherapy in England in 1995 and has been in practice ever since. He practises at the Atman Clinic in Tunbridge Wells. In addition to seeing patients, Peter is involved in several other areas of herbal activity including education and professional regulation. Peter views herbal medicine as both an ancient art and a modern science. His work is founded on understanding herbal medicine by integrating the perspectives of rational evidence-based medicine, traditional herbal writings and the knowledge gained from clinical experience. He passionately believes that herbal medicine should and will emerge as an important strand of mainstream medicine during the twenty-first century.

Charles Cunningham

Charles Cunningham is a qualified Health Advisor in Maharishi Ayurveda. He has a BSc in psychology and an MSc in health promotion for which he conducted empirical research on tridosha theory. In 2000, he published in the *American Journal of Cardiology* a study conducted at St George's Hospital on the effects of Transcendental Meditation on a heart condition known as cardiac syndrome X. Charles has also taught Transcendental Meditation to more than 2000 people over 15 years, and has lectured on this and Ayurveda to doctors, university audiences, conferences and adult education courses. Previously, Charles was a Senior Database Analyst in the IT industry.

Alison Denham

Alison has been in practice in Leeds as a herbal practitioner since qualifying as a Member of the National Institute of Medical Herbalists (NIMH) in 1984. She was Director of Research of NIMH 1998–2000 and then its President 2000–2002. She represented the National Institute on the Herbal Medicine Regulatory Working Group. She has been a part-time Senior Lecturer in Herbal Medicine on the degree programme at the University of Central Lancashire since 2000, teaching Materia Medica and Herbal Pharmacology, Herbal Pharmacy, Therapeutics in Herbal Medicine and Clinical Audit. Her research interests include: pilot randomized controlled study into the treatment of menopausal complaints by herbal practitioners, clinical audit, safety of medicinal plants. Other interests: conservation and cultivation of North American medicinal plants.

Katia Holmes

Katia Holmes gained an MA in political science at SciencePo in Paris and went on to gain an MSc in economics at the University of Paris, where she then taught. Since 1971, she has devoted her life to the preservation of Tibetan culture and in particular to the translation of its literature. She studied traditional Tibetan medicine under Professor Khenpo Troru Tsenam, the leading physician in present-day Tibet, from 1994 onwards during a series of six yearly teaching visits to Scotland and interpreted for him and other Tibetan doctors and also taught part of the course herself.

Peter Jackson-Main

Peter Jackson-Main was born in London in 1955 and began his study of alternative and complementary medicine shortly after gaining his degree at Cambridge University in 1977. He is qualified in Herbal Medicine, Iridology, Polarity Therapy and Core Energetic Therapy. He has been instrumental in establishing two professional associations, the Polarity Therapy Association of the UK, and the Association of Master Herbalists (UK), of which he is currently chairman. He is also secretary of the European Herbal Practitioners Association and has been closely involved in the political processes surrounding herbal medicine since 1994.

Nick Lampert

Nick Lampert started professional life in social sciences at the University of Birmingham. He left in 1989 to study Chinese medicine, firstly acupuncture (London School of Acupuncture and Traditional Chinese Medicine, graduated 1992), and then, later, Chinese herbal medicine (School of Chinese Herbal Medicine, graduated 1996). He obtained further clinical training in Nanjing, China in 1992 (acupuncture) and in 1996 (herbal medicine). In 1995, Nick joined two colleagues to set up the Birmingham Centre for Chinese Medicine, where he now practises herbal medicine and acupuncture in about equal proportions. He is a former Chair of the Register of Chinese Herbal Medicine, and represented the RCHM on the Herbal Medicine Regulatory Working Group.

Michael McIntyre

Michael McIntyre is Chair of the European Herbal Practitioners Association. He practises Chinese and western herbal medicine and acupuncture in his clinic in the Cotswolds. He is author of two books and many articles on herbal medicine and broadcasts regularly on the subject. He is also a Trustee of the Prince of Wales Foundation for Integrated Health and an external examiner for Chinese and Western herbal medicine at the University of Westminster.

Catherine O'Sullivan

Catherine O'Sullivan has served as Chair of the Education Committee of the EHPA since her time as Principal of the Northern College of Acupuncture. She has worked at Leeds Metropolitan University and Newman College of Higher Education, where she was Vice-Principal. Her research interest is in education for professional practice, and she has taught in the field of leadership and management. Her latest role is with Birmingham and the Black Country Strategic Health Authority, where she has responsibility for workforce education and learning.

Victoria Pitman

Victoria Pitman comes from the United States and first graduated in English and, with an MA in Teaching, began a teaching career in secondary education. In the 1980s she trained in herbal medicine and bodywork and entered clinical practice. She is a tutor and lecturer in herbal medicine, aromatherapy and reflexology and has authored articles in professional journals. Vicki is a member of the United Register of Herbal Practitioners, the American Herbalists Guild and the International Federation of Aromatherapists and Association of Reflexologists. An interest in the history of herbal medicine led her to research its foundations in the ancient world and to undertake an MPhil in Complementary Health Studies at the University of Exeter, on which her chapter in this present volume is based. The dissertation was published in late 2004 as *Sources of holism in Ancient Greek and Indian medicine*.

R Michael Pittilo

Professor Mike Pittilo has been Pro Vice-Chancellor at the University of Hertfordshire since 2002. Prior to this he was Dean of Health and Social Care Sciences at Kingston University and St George's Hospital Medical School (University of London) and Dean for postgraduate taught courses at the Medical School. He was chair of the Herbal Medicine Regulatory Working Group and currently chairs the Quality Assurance Agency for the Higher Education Benchmarking Group for the Health Professions as well as being a Non-Executive Director of the NHS Bedfordshire and Hertfordshire Health Authority. He is a biologist with research interests in parasitology and vascular endothelium.

Brion Sweeney

Brion Sweeney trained as a family physician and is a member of the Royal College of Psychiatrists (1983) with a Masters degree in psychotherapy. He has taken a special interest in Eastern approaches to the mind and offers psychotherapeutic approaches using Eastern and Western approaches. He is Clinical Director of Addiction Services for the Northern Area Health Board (population 0.5 M) of the Eastern Regional Authority in Ireland.

Foreword

CLARENCE HOUSE

I am delighted to introduce this book, which marks an important stage in the development of integrated healthcare in the U.K. Principally, it seeks to explore some of the complexities associated with using traditional knowledge in modern healthcare settings, and with the potential gains to patients that can be offered by extending choice within our National Health Service. At the same time, the book recognizes the impact for practitioners associated with a change in their professional status as integrated care advancers,and discusses some of the tensions that this may bring for the practitioner community. Whilst the subject of this book is herbal medicine, its themes will be of enormous relevance to all those who have an interest in integrated healthcare, be it professional or personal.

As far as I am concerned, the vision I have for integrated health is all about combining the best of the ancient with the best of the modern. Integrated healthcare is not just about complementary medicine, nor is it a substitute for conventional care. Rather, it is about understanding that, in the complex world of the twenty-first century, no single therapeutic strategy, and no one approach to knowledge, can have a monopoly on effective diagnosis and treatment for all conditions. Scientific, psychological, nutritional, environmental and spiritual insights all have a role in maintaining and restoring health and wellbeing. An integrated approach offers different therapeutic options, supporting patient choice, and with the additional benefit of delivering huge potential cost savings in the management of chronic long-term sickness.

My Foundation for Integrated Health is dedicated to the development of safe and effective integrated healthcare in the United Kingdom. It has worked with the herbal community since its inception to support the development of the case for statutory self-regulation and the move to make herbal medicine more widely available throughout the UK and the Western world. Over this time, I have seen very real progress being made. There is increased use by the public of herbal products, greater co-operation between herbalists and conventional practitioners and considerable progress towards regulation – the background to this book. Naturally enough, this development has created a considerable amount of controversy, debate and dialogue. I am delighted that an account of the move towards the statutory regulation of herbal practitioners, highlighting the fundamental issues involved, is being made available through this work.

The demand for herbal medicines has another aspect. At a time when farmers everywhere are struggling to make ends meet, the development of a natural pharmacy of organically grown herbs offers an alternative means of earning a living. However, we need to ensure that modern farming methods, deforestation in Asia and the Amazon and the effects of globalization on small farmers in India are not allowed to continue to threaten traditional herbal crops, and the families and communities who depend on them, at the very time when Western medical science is beginning to recognize their benefits. That is where the knowledge base of the different herbal traditions represented in this publication has much to offer modern agriculture, as well as to healthcare.

I hope that this book will stimulate innovation in the ways we think about medicine and healthcare practice, so that patients can benefit from the true integration of the best of complementary and orthodox medical approaches, for the maintenance and enhancement of their health and well-being.

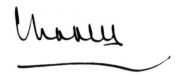

Acknowledgements

We shall not cease from exploration
And the end of all our exploring
Will be to arrive where we started
And know the place for the first time.
(T. S. Eliot, Little Gidding V, *Four Quartets*, 1943)

THANKS ARE DUE TO:

Amrit Ahluwalia, Project Director of the European Herbal Practitioners Association and stalwart Secretary to the Herbal Medicine Regulatory Working Group;

Lynn Copcutt, and all the Education Committee and Accreditation Board of the EHPA, for their hard work and enthusiasm;

The Prince of Wales, and the staff of his Foundation for Integrated Health;

All civil servants in the Department of Health and the Medicines and Healthcare Products Regulatory Agency, who have worked towards legislation that protects the freedoms of herbalists;

Pamela Taylor, Principal of Newman College of Higher Education, and all employers who support professional development activity;

Eva-Maria Lenz, for invaluable help with the manuscript;

Terry, Tom, Isabelle, Oliver, Ruari and Ned O'Sullivan, and all our families who tolerate our unexplained absences on urgent business elsewhere.

List of abbreviations

AMA	Ayurvedic Medical Association
AMH	Association of Master Herbalists
ARWG	Acupuncture Regulatory Working Group
ATCM	Association of Traditional Chinese Medicine
BAAAP	British Association of Accredited Ayurvedic Practitioners
BAMC	British Ayurvedic Medical Council
BATTM	British Association of Traditional Tibetan Medicine
BHMA	British Herbal Medicine Association
BSCM	British Society of Chinese Medicine
CAM	Complementary and alternative medicine
CCAM	Council for Complementary and Alternative Medicine
CPD	Continuing professional development
CPMP	Committee on Proprietary Medicinal Products
CPP	College of Practitioners of Phytotherapy
CRHP	Council for the Regulation of Healthcare Professionals
DH	Department of Health
DTHMP	Directive on Traditional Herbal Medicinal Products
EBM	Evidence-based medicine
EHPA	European Herbal Practitioners Association
EMEA	European Medicines Evaluation Agency
GMC	General Medical Council
GMP	Good Manufacturing Practice
HMRWG	Herbal Medicine Regulatory Working Group
HPC	Health Professions Council
IMB	Irish Medicines Board
IRCH	International Register of Consultant Herbalists
MAPA	Maharishi Ayurveda Practitioners Association
MAV	Maharishi Ayurveda
MCA	Medicines Control Agency
MHRA	Medicines and Healthcare Products Regulatory Agency
NHS	National Health Service
NIMH	National Institute of Medical Herbalists
NPU	National Poisons Unit
OTC	Over the counter
PA	Pyrrolizidine alkaloid
PoWFIH	Prince of Wales's Foundation for Integrated Health
RCHM	Register of Chinese Herbal Medicine
RCT	Randomized controlled trials
RPSGB	Royal Pharmaceutical Society of Great Britain
SSR	Statutory self-regulation
TCM	Traditional Chinese medicine

TM	Transcendental Meditation
TTM	Traditional Tibetan Medicine
UKCC	United Kingdom Central Council for Nursing, Midwifery and Health Visiting
URHP	Unified Register of Herbal Practitioners
WHO	World Health Organization

Introduction
Reshaping herbal medicine: the context

Catherine O'Sullivan

This book is about herbal medicine. It is about what herbalists do, the herbal products they use, and the way that the profession and the practice are evolving in a wider process of evolution, and revolution, in the delivery of health services. Beyond that, the book is concerned with the place of alternative and complementary medicine within a society dominated by a rational and scientific approach to illness, which privileges the treatment of illness over the health and well-being of a whole person.

This book arose from a series of protracted, and often contentious, debates among a loosely knit group of herbal practitioners and their professional associates around the case for statutory self-regulation. In determining the way forward in the UK, and in seeking to build consensus within sceptical groupings of practitioners, many different commentators were drawn into wide-ranging debates around what it means to be a professional. These could be styled as a series of 'reflective conversations' around knowledge and professional culture, and the ways in which a sense of collective norms are developed within a professional community, or communities. At the point at which specific proposals on potential legislation were published by the UK Department of Health, it seemed a good idea to share some of these debates beyond those who had been involved initially, including those colleagues overseas who are examining these issues themselves within their local healthcare systems.

Through an examination of the emergence of the profession of herbalist, a theme hitherto not examined in any of the literature on healthcare professions, *Reshaping Herbal Medicine* offers unique and important insights into the development of professional identity.

In challenging the dominant model of healthcare in the West, each of the contributors offers personal insights into alternative ways of thinking about health and ill health. Drawing on the rich traditions that inform their own practice, the contributors are interested in an examination of the ways in which traditional forms of practice coexist alongside more modern understandings of medical treatment. This book is not a clinical textbook. It is rather a discussion about the integration of different forms of medicine in a complex, industrialized economy with a diverse and ageing population. What more can be added to what is already available, and how does this further the interest of patients?

Put more formally, the purpose of the book is to investigate some of the implicit principles and concepts that are influencing the move towards the statutory self-regulation (SSR) of herbal medicine.

Its aims are:

- to explore the concept of the healthcare professional in relation to the emergent profession of (medical) herbalist
- to discuss some of the problems of integration into mainstream structures, including the gains and losses to the practitioner community
- to describe aspects of the different traditions that make up the practice of herbal medicine, and to make links and comparisons between them
- to debate the ways in which traditional knowledge, and the knowledge that is known in expert practice, can be shared, communicated and critiqued within the notion of an evidence base for clinical efficacy
- to question some aspects of current policy in relation to patient care and a national health service, and suggest some ways in which herbal medicine can make a distinctive contribution.

In order to achieve these aims, the book uses material drawn from the last 10 years in the UK, and beyond across Europe. The recent history of the use of herbal products shows both a growth in the public use of natural medicines and threats to patient safety from poor advice and inadequate quality control. This has impacted on that group of practitioners who have undergone a formal training in herbal medicine; as have other, wider, changes in the structures of modern society. The impact of these changes is for that group of practitioners (those who are formally trained) to come together and, collectively, ask themselves whether or not they can be construed as being a single profession. What are the implications of developing a shared professional identity for those who come together from such diverse backgrounds? What would be the boundaries of professional practice for those who might use herbal medicines alongside other therapeutic practices, such as massage or acupuncture? What kinds of behaviours would be associated with a common professional identity, and would any of these challenge traditional practices, which date back many centuries, and which originated from cultures very different to modern Europe?

The historical process that forms the context of this book, the move towards the statutory self-regulation of the herbal profession, spans a 10-year period. Chapter 9 gives more detail of the recent history in the UK and Europe. Throughout this period, the above questions have formed an implicit background to all the developments. The purpose of the present work is to make this debate explicit, and to frame it against a more theoretical examination of the nature of professional identity. A number of substantive issues emerge from the debate.

A first key area of difficulty is around the nature of knowledge, and of the kinds of knowledge that are embedded in a clinical discipline. Who defines what constitutes acceptable knowledge, and what epistemological and methodological assumptions underpin the ideas of medicine? In the case of traditional medicine, there are particular cultural sensitivities to be noted. On the one hand, it can be argued that the positivist approach that underpins much of Western scientific medicine is a Eurocentric model, which fails to respect other ways of thinking about knowledge. Traditional Chinese Medicine (TCM) and Ayurvedic medicine are scholarly traditions, based on written texts, and on centuries of empirical evidence drawn from multiple documented case studies. There have been 'schools' of medicine established throughout Asia for many centuries, which have originated, validated and transmitted such knowledge often through an 'apprentice/master' model of professional education. Although such methods differ from modern practices, they are not necessarily less rigorous or less effective in terms of professional formation. Similarly, in the Western traditions, there have been a number of established groupings of practitioners, some of which have belonged in formal collective agreements for voluntary registration for over a hundred years (Chapter 6).

On the other hand, in looking at forms of knowledge with their roots in ancient cultures, there is also a risk that such knowledge will be appropriated without the understanding or the consent of minority communities, who now represent such cultures in the West. In this sense, many Western herbal practitioners would also see themselves as a minority culture, drawing as they do on ways of knowing that are rather different to the dominant biomedical model of healthcare. Nevertheless, they argue that their knowledge is clinically based, consisting of empirical findings, which are contained in written texts and transmitted through both formal schools and more informal, personal, teacher/student relationships. Appropriation could stem from a popularizing of ancient ways of knowing, through a zeitgeist that commodifies cultural arte-facts and sells them as fashion accessories. Or it could arise from the commer-cial interest of pharmaceutical companies, who look to identify and patent the active ingredients in some plant medicines, without considering the impact on the communities who have never protected their traditional knowledge. Or knowledge could be appropriated by other healthcare professionals, who add a treatment modality to their own form of practice without understanding the theory base of the system of medicine from which such a practice emerges. All of these forms of cultural appropriation represent a threat to any emergent profession of herbalist.

A second area of difficulty, in debates around the formation of professional identity, is in respect of the relationship with the patient within the clinical encounter. Here, the difficulty mainly lies in relation to the emphasis on the centrality of patient safety to the whole debate on practitioner identity. While the rhetoric of all healthcare practitioners will always place patient safety at the heart of any debate, the reality can be somewhat different. Very real difficulties have emerged over the potential risks and benefits to patients from some of the herbal products in use over the 10-year period upon which this book draws. This related in some instances to products sold over the counter in healthfood shops, and sometimes to concerns over products that arose in other countries. An instance of this is kava kava in Germany. The scientific evidence was ambiguous, with practitioners being of the view that some of the perceived changes arose from the use of modern manufacturing processes, in preference to the traditional ways of preparing, prescribing and dispensing herbs (see, for example, Chapter 5).

In relation to the nature of the service offered to patients, there were also some conflicts around patient safety and patient choice. In some parts of our society, herbal remedies have been the treatment of choice for particular groups, who were poorer or whose background led them to a particular kind of therapist. In formalizing and regulating the profession in terms of patient safety, might there be some unexpected consequences in terms of patient choice for some of the more marginalized groups in our society?

Part of the problem here has related to the lack of detailed understanding about motivation and patient choice. Through the process of building the case for statutory self-regulation, there has been a greater involvement of lay people in the work of the professional bodies and practitioner associations. But do such lay people really represent the patients' interest, or is their role rather to protect the dominant ideologies of state-funded healthcare or higher education?

The third area of difficulty for the practitioners who were developing into a profession relates to the balance of autonomy and independence with integration into the mainstream. Historically, some of the practitioner associations had a long pedigree, and had seen themselves as 'alternative' to the national provision of healthcare. There were great difficulties for many individual practitioners, and for some professional bodies, about working with other traditions on a road that was intended to lead towards a statutorily defined place in the healthcare service of the UK and Europe. In the working lives of such practitioners, over a relatively short period there seemed to have been a move from 'alternative' to 'complementary' to 'integrated'. Even such language, implying some sort of positioning vis-à-vis the orthodoxy, causes difficulty to some.

Equally, for others, an accommodation with the mainstream structures represents the only way that herbal practice could survive. Others again felt that full integration into the NHS would lead to a growth and blossoming of herbal medicine in ways that have not been seen in Europe for many centuries, with a consequential positive impact on the health of many thousands of patients. These differing perspectives all contributed to the complexities of the debate around the proposed changes.

Because medical law is framed at the European level, and yet the regulation of professions remains part of national law, it was possible to envisage different ways of framing the problems and identifying solutions. This, at times, has led to considerable conflict among practitioner groups as different positions emerged from rather different implicit models of professional regulation. Even when accepting the necessity, or benefits, of some sense of collective professional identity that was formalized and recognized by the state, there were different options in terms of scope and degree. Should regulation be statutory or voluntary? Should it regulate for entry into the profession, for the codes of ethics that determine practice, or for the products that can or cannot be used? These were vexed questions, which went to the heart of individual practitioners' personal sense of their role and their status.

This book has grown out of the 10-year period during which these kinds of problems were debated, discussed, defined and then disseminated to the wider public. All of the contributors to the book have been involved in this process for several years, and have played a personal role in the evolution of professional identity for herbal medicine, at this particular historic moment.

The editor and the contributors have all been associated with the European Herbal Practitioners Association, one of the three stakeholders (together with the Department of Health and the Prince of Wales's Foundation for Integrated Health) to the Herbal Medicine Regulatory Working Group. It is from the process of developing the recommendations of that group (Herbal Medicine Regulatory Working Group 2003) that this book is drawn. All of the contributors are either practising herbalists, or are involved in working and researching in higher education, or both. This book draws upon their diverse and extensive expertise in the development of herbal medicine, and in the professional formation of herbalists.

An examination of the emergence of the profession of herbalist, a theme hitherto not examined in any of the literature on healthcare professions, offers unique and important insights into the development of professional identity. The work is characterized by an unusually tight collaboration between the contributors, as the profession prepares itself for major change. Each chapter of the book has been informed by the wider landscape, and by the relationship of each distinctive contribution to the overall process of statutory self-regulation. For this reason, the book is presented in three sections, to allow individual readers to select the content most relevant to their interest. The first section is concerned with the nature of professions, the second with the traditions of herbal medicine, and the third with the problems of the current proposed changes.

The book starts with a theoretical section, which offers an overview of the literature on professions. This was shared among all contributors, as an agreed framework against which the problems of professional identity in the herbal community could be examined. Many of these ideas were actively discussed throughout the years during which the background work was being done, to prepare the case for a claim under the Health Act 1999 to be recognized as a profession. As part of the preparation of the case, a large number of policy documents had to be written, particularly in relation to the education of practitioners who would be eligible to be called herbalists. The development of such policy needed to be underpinned by an understanding of the distinctive markers of professional identity.

The next section of the book considers the four main traditions of herbal medicine that are being brought together into the proposed new statutory body. In describing the traditions for readers who are not familiar with them, the authors of these traditions also consider the salient features of the tradition at this historical point in time, and how those features will accommodate themselves to a new context.

Chapter 3, the first chapter in this middle section, is concerned with TCM. In discussing the evolution of Chinese medicine across the world, and more recently in the UK, Nick Lampert addresses the issue of 'what is the nature of practice?' He begins by outlining some of the diagnostic concepts and approaches, before considering the treatment options. There are particularly complex issues around Chinese medicine, in terms of the relationship between herbal practice and the main other modality, acupuncture. The random effects of history have led to the situation in the UK where the practice of acupuncture, in particular, can be separated from the underpinning knowledge that is known as TCM. The strong wish of the Chinese herbal community in Britain is for TCM to be regulated as a whole.

Katia Holmes examines the history of Tibetan medicine in Chapter 4. Of the four traditions, this is the least well known in the UK and Europe. However, perhaps because of Tibet's own recent history, there is a great wish in its country of origin to support the wider knowledge and practice of Tibetan herbal medicine in other countries of the world. Katia examines in this chapter the ways that different small subgroupings came together to work within the process on offer in the UK to ensure that this ancient tradition, although not yet well known outside Asia, is recognized as a tradition within its own right.

In Chapter 5, Charles Cunningham gives an historical account of the development of Ayurvedic medicine. He is concerned to emphasize the ways in which Ayurvedic medicine has always been a scholarly tradition, learning from and contributing to other great medical systems. For this reason, Ayurvedic and Western medicine are practised in an integrated way in India. This offers a successful model of integration to Western countries.

Chapter 6, by Peter Jackson-Main, is concerned with Western herbal medicine and explores the issues from a somewhat different perspective to the chapters that precede it. The issue in terms of Western herbal medicine is not to familiarize a Western reader to a system of medicine that is strange to them. Rather, it is to ask why the indigenous practice became so marginalized within our society. Peter offers several answers, as does Michael McIntyre later on in Chapter 9. Among the issues Peter addresses, with his co-contributor Julie Cox, is a gendered reading of the history of herbal medicine, which associates herbs and simples with women. It can be argued that to read the history of herbal medicine in the UK is to read the history of women in Britain. However, there are other forces at work, and Peter also questions the dangers of basing professional identity too closely on the orthodox idea of a doctor as the paradigm for a professional.

In the last chapter in this section, Chapter 7, Victoria Pitman also examines Western herbal medicine. However, her discussion is less concerned with the history of the evolution of herbal medicine in the UK than with examining the classical sources from which such a tradition is derived. She questions why contemporary herbalists in the Western tradition have lost touch with the ancient scholarship that underpins their history, in contrast to her Chinese, Tibetan and Ayurvedic contemporaries, who are still knowledgeable about the ancient texts of their traditions. In rediscovering the Hippocratic corpus, Vicky rediscovers the Greek understanding of the concept of *holism*, a concept central to today's practitioners. The question raised by Vicky in this chapter, in relation to the philosophy of medical knowledge which informs her own contemporary practice, points the way to the final section of the book in relation to its questioning of how knowledge is developed, transmitted, owned or lost.

The third section of the book explores five of the key themes that emerged as significant in the examination of the case for the statutory self-regulation of herbal medicine. Each of these themes is presented in terms of its problems, and set within a series of wider debates around professional identity. There are clear areas of overlap within the themes, but with different perspectives on how to resolve the areas of difficulty, depending on whose interest is being considered: the practitioner, the patient or the wider public good. This last section attempts to transcend the confines of the situation in the UK to examine some universal themes of relevance to any reader with an interest in professional knowledge and culture.

Chapter 8, by Michael Pittilo, looks at the place of herbal medicine within the wider framework of the National Health Service (NHS) reforms. With patient safety being seen by Mike as the central driving force behind the proposed changes, he argues that only a statutorily regulated profession will give patients the protection that they should expect. In discussing the form that such regulation should take, Mike argues in effect that herbal medicine cannot be taken seriously as a profession if it eschews the forms adopted by the well-established professions already in existence. To allow self-interest or the protectionism of special interest groups to dominate the agenda is to deny the herbal profession credibility with the wider public.

Michael McIntyre, in Chapter 9, has a different perspective on the political forces that are driving change. His analysis places UK legislation lower, in the hierarchy of external influences on professional identity, than the potential threat to herbal medicines that arises from the European context. His endpoint echoes that of Mike above, as he argues that only a fully regulated profession will ensure the survival of herbs as medical products, to the long-term benefits of patients. His colourful account of the battle of herbalists to win their place among the state-recognized healthcare professions documents the difficulties that have been encountered, both within and outside the profession.

Nick Lampert makes a second contribution to the book, in his discussion of culture and knowledge in relation to herbal medicine, in Chapter 10. His concern is with the ways in which traditional knowledge, and traditional ways of knowing embedded in clinical practice, can be maintained and extended in the post-SSR world. How is Chinese medicine to relate to Western orthodoxy, and which strategies will best ensure that the practice of TCM retains its vitality while moving towards the goal of integrated healthcare? His answer is to be found in a conceptualization of heterogeneity, where Chinese and Western medicine exist alongside each other, with a dialogue between the two systems that allows for multiplicity in practice and openness to change. In advocating this approach, Nick is not blind to the difficulties this will bring in practice, and to the inequalities in the exchanges between the two systems.

Alison Denham, in Chapter 11, grapples with many of the same issues in her discussion on education and the professional formation of herbal practitioners. From her experiences, she analyses the difficulties in meeting both the general requirements of the academic infrastructure (subject benchmarks and so on) and the particular requirements of a preparation for practice as a herbalist. Balancing the necessary theoretical knowledge with the acquisition of skills is a challenge in all programmes of professional education, but it is exacerbated for herbal medicine because of the tensions between scientific and holistic ways of viewing the clinical encounter. These tensions arise in part from the differences between higher education and the professional bodies in terms of their ideas about knowledge, and in part from disagreements between different professional associations themselves about the relative weight of different elements in the curriculum.

Knowledge is again the issue in the last chapter, Chapter 12, contributed by Peter Conway. His concern, echoing some of the areas highlighted earlier by Nick and Alison, is with the nature of knowledge itself and the difficulty of meaningful dialogue with different interest groups when their epistemological understandings remain relatively underexamined. For herbalists, coming together to discuss the nature of professional identity in their preparation of the case for the statutory self-regulation of herbal medicine, the debate has endlessly focused and refocused on the same group of core problems. Why are we seeking self-regulation? Is it really to protect the public, and to develop our understanding of what we do so that we can help our patients more effectively?

And do we serve our client group better if we remain independent, focusing our efforts on the development of our own practice, and undistracted by engagements with the wide range of other agencies that make up the state health and education systems? Or do we risk losing all that is special to us if we remain aloof from the rest of civil society, and we lose the trust of our patients?

The contributors in this book, including the editor, have all had to examine aspects of these problems as policy developed in relation to education and continuing professional development (CPD), codes of ethics and practice, processes to assure the quality of both the education of practitioners and the manufacture of products, and systems and structures that support different potential models of regulation. In developing such policy, core ideas and concepts have had to be explained to, and explored and questioned by, a very diverse group of commentators, ranging from politicians and the media, to groups of practitioners and individual herbalists, to such other statutory bodies as the Quality Assurance Agency or the Medicines and Healthcare Products Regulatory Agency. This debate has happened in the four countries of the UK, in Ireland, in other European countries and in Brussels, with the agencies of the EU.

In developing the ideas that are conceptualized and presented as problems in the present volume, the contributors are drawing on all this work: from memory, from formal records and documents and from other professional activities of theirs that supported their policy roles. This raises some interesting methodological issues, with which I wish to conclude this introduction.

The methodological concerns are in relation to authenticity, rigour and stance.

In terms of authenticity, the account of the process in this volume is informed by the personal participation of all contributors. They (we) have had access to a wide variety of times and places in which these ideas have been formulated, and have had access to the various drafts of policy documents as they have been drafted and redrafted. This gives the unique perspective of the participant.

The weakness of this approach is the lack of critical detachment from the situation that is offered by the independent researcher. To some extent, this has been counteracted by the involvement of others in the development of the different chapters, making their own contributions and acting as critical readers. Nevertheless, the collection of essays offered here are not representative of the views of either the practitioner community or of a detached researcher. They are written from a position of commitment, from individuals who have chosen to give up their time and energy because they believe in the idea of a unified herbal profession that is recognized as part of the official healthcare system in the four countries of the UK.

It is important that readers of this book recognize the authenticity of the authorial voices, and their concomitant position as actors in a political and historical process. Associated with the potential bias of the committed position of the authors is the question of rigour. Rigour, in interpretative research, is usually conveyed by triangulating emergent understandings with other examples of the same issue, looking particularly for disconfirming instances. It is from this kind of a process that this present work evolves. The product of the work around the development of the case for statutory self-regulation was the report of the Regulatory Working Group (Herbal Medicine Regulatory Working Group 2003). This was itself the culmination of several earlier years of policy formation and development. In reaching its conclusion and recommendations, the Regulatory Working Group took evidence from, and consulted with, a very wide group of individuals and bodies.

In formulating its views, the Herbal Medicine Regulatory Working Group engaged in considerable consultation and debate. The involvement of the contributors in such a breadth of views, often expressed very strongly, has tested the acceptability of some of the policy to the practitioner community. Such testing of ideas over an extended period of time can be seen to provide a triangulating function to this present work. All of the contributors, on occasion, have found themselves turning back to re-examine some personal position, in a reflexive revisiting of central constructs. Often, the settled has become contested again, by a different group or when the context appears to change. This has led us to identify some inherent contradictions between principles and the deliverables of pragmatism and political reality.

It is the problems and difficulties that emerged from this process that are being discussed in this present work. Even so, in order to make the account coherent, there has been an incredible amount of 'tidying up' of the narrative, in order to convey some central ideas to a variety of potential readers. This has inevitably led to some oversimplifications of complex debates, perhaps also leading to some marginalization of minority dissenting positions. This difficulty has to be acknowledged as part of the process of communicating a multifaceted approach, over a long period, to a number of problems around professional identity.

Finally, the question of stance requires some brief exploration. The stance of the contributors to this book has been acknowledged above, as a group of actors in a real-world process who have worked together and co-constructed some concepts around professional identity in relation to herbal medicine. In acknowledging this stance, we invite readers also to consider their position as the audience to this work.

We envisage three groups of readers for this book. The first group, perhaps the nearest to our own interest, is that of the practitioner community. They should see their own views represented here, but may take exception to some of the conclusions that are drawn. Practitioners are affected by the changes that are in train, and cannot detach their own sense of self-identity from any conceptualization of the herbal practitioner from a given tradition.

A very different sort of reader is the general reader, who may be using this book to gain an overview of herbal medicine, perhaps with a view to using herbs as medicines, or perhaps with a more general interest in alternative and complementary medicine. Such readers may find the contributors overly concerned with the story of where all this began, not realizing the extent to which history has shaped the present moment, in the minds of the practitioner community. For such readers, the interest in this volume may rest rather more in the discussion of the place of herbal medicine within the structures of society than in the difficulties such a transition makes for the professional herbalist.

Thirdly, it is anticipated that this book will be read by a variety of different kinds of non-herbal practitioners, both in complementary and in orthodox healthcare professions, and by academic readers concerned with professional education. For such an audience, the interest of the book may reside in the ways in which practitioners see their relationships developing with others, particularly in terms of the extension of knowledge. Some of the difficulties experienced by practitioners may seem self-indulgent in the context of delivering greater patient choice and enhanced patient safety. At the same time, such readers may want to consider aspects of their own sense of professional identity by taking up a personal position in relation to some of the more problematic areas treated by the book.

The danger with writing a book like this is that it fails to transcend the particular situation, in order to present overarching concepts that can be explored outside the historical context in which the concepts are grounded. There are contradictions and confusions present in this volume; this represents our perception of the complexity of the agenda with which we are working. As editor, it is my hope that, if you can select from within the contributions in this book those themes that have most salience for you, you will share some of the intellectual excitement that has been generated for us along the journey.

References

Herbal Medicine Regulatory Working Group 2003 Recommendations on the Regulation of Herbal Practitioners in the UK. Prince of Wales's Foundation for Integrated Health, London

Knowledge, education and professional culture

1

Determining professional identity:

an exploration of the factors that characterize the nature of a profession

Catherine O'Sullivan

OVERVIEW

The purpose of the collection of essays in this volume is to consider the ways in which professional identity is being manifested and determined in herbal medicine during the time of working towards statutory self-regulation, or SSR (currently anticipated to take place in 2006). It will be argued that the changes incumbent upon herbalists are redefining their own sense of what it means to become a professional. Such changes, at the level of the practitioner, include relationships with patients, working with other professionals and a more formal requirement for professional updating. For the profession as a whole, the move to SSR has consequences for initial education, the definition of an acceptable evidence base, the structures that support regulation and the need to legitimize relationships with a whole range of other bodies, not least the Department of Health (DH).

The purpose of this chapter and the next is therefore to set these debates into a theoretical context. Before considering in detail the implications of changes in professional identity for herbalists, it is necessary first to examine the ways in which professions are formed, developed and change.

CONCEPTUALIZING THE PROFESSIONAL

Eraut (1994, p. 223) raises some interesting questions about the ideological nature of professions. In this analysis, he suggests that there are three distinct characteristics of professions that correspond to an ideal. These are:

- a specialist knowledge base
- autonomy or independence in the exercise of judgement
- the delivery of a distinctive service to a client group, with an attendant ethical responsibility to them.

These three concepts are key to this study of the recent evolution of the profession of herbal medicine. Each of the chapters in Section Three will explore the problematic aspects of these interrelated dimensions.

Each of these concepts can also be viewed as interesting and complex for any given profession and, as this chapter will seek to demonstrate, this is no less the case for herbal medicine:

"Like all effective ideologies, the ideology of professionalism embodies appealing values, in this case those of service, trustworthiness, integrity, autonomy and reliable standards; it works in the interests of certain groups – those occupations recognized as professions – while winning the consent, most of the time, of others whose interests are less certainly served by it; and it is effective in so far as its representation of reality is accepted as obviously correct."

(McIntyre 1994, p. viii)

Eraut (1994) focuses on these three distinct areas of professional identity both as defining features and as aspects of professionalism that he feels require further critical examination. He and other commentators (Becher 1999a, Downie 1990, Thompson 1997) argue that the nature of professions and professional identity is highly problematic at present, and under threat from a number of different influences. The very fact that professional identity may seem to be threatened is likely to result in professions laying a greater emphasis than hitherto on the defining characteristics of their particular professional grouping. Such threats are likely to reinforce the status quo, and to create a defensive and guarded response to new developments in interdisciplinary workings (McNeill 1999, Whitty 1999). The drive to regulate herbal medicine is, in part, a defensive reaction to prevent the extensive use of herbal products by other, unqualified, professionals.

Eraut (1994) suggests that, towards the end of the twentieth century, the distinctiveness of the professional knowledge base became complex and multidimensional. Complexity is a response to the growth in specializations and the interdependency of professionals who operate in multiagency ways. Such changes coincide with a development of critiques of the ways in which professions develop their knowledge.

So it is also with regard to the concept of professional autonomy. Eraut (1994) discusses two ways in which the greater emphasis on professional accountability is acting as a driver for change in the ways professions perceive themselves and are perceived. These are, first, the scrutiny now being directed at the structure of the ways in which professions regulate themselves, and, secondly, a reduction in the individual practitioner's personal autonomy and responsibility for the exercising of professional judgement. This latter he discusses in the context of practitioners who are employed by organizations, and who therefore may experience some tensions between organizational goals and controls and their own autonomous practice. This might occur, for example, in large NHS trusts.

Finally, Eraut suggests that, traditionally, professional notions of the service ideal were predicated on the belief that professional action should be based on the needs of the client alone, and not on the needs of the professional or of society as a whole. He sees the service ideal also as under threat from such concepts as client rights and client choice, which remove the assumption that professionals know what is best for the client by virtue of their superior knowledge. He sees further difficulties with defining *who* is the client in some of the settings in which professional services are delivered. In multiagency care settings, for example, there can be many stakeholders to whom some sort of professional service is due.

Eraut's analysis establishes a context of change, to which can be added one further change agent: the pace of professional change, fuelled by technology and scientific discovery, is blurring distinctions between the needs of clients and the wider interests of society. (This is seen, for example, with biomedical advances in genetics or the treatment of infertility, where clinicians make decisions that may set precedents for others in the field.) Increasingly, professionals are required to balance the needs of the client with wider ethical concerns that may not yet have been debated or agreed within society. This places a greater burden on the individual professional, who may be at the forefront of new practice and thus be placed in the position of discriminating between the conflicting interests of different groups.

In summary, in all of these areas, there is a greater emphasis on outcomes than was ever the case before. This emphasis is fundamentally changing the very nature of professional practice. The impact of these changes will differentially affect different professions. However, in all professions their impact is likely to be seen on the values that underpin practice, the ways that capability to practice is developed over the lifetime of the professional, and in the ways more public knowledge is developed and disseminated (Barnett 1994, Downie 1990). There is a dynamic and shifting relationship between these three aspects of professionalism. Becher (1999a, p. 3) suggests that:

"studies of professional values could be given a clearer focus if viewed against a background of change: and that the strategies involved to cope with such change would throw light on the process of maintaining professional knowledge and capability."

This study is concerned with developing an understanding of the distinctive nature of professional knowledge and expertise for the practitioner of herbal medicine at a period of change and development for the profession. It seeks to understand the ways professional characteristics can be defined, developed or distorted by the processes of professional regulation and education.

WHAT IS A PROFESSION?

In examining the case study of an emergent profession, it is necessary first to consider what is meant by the term 'profession'. There is an extensive literature on professions, which suggests that agreeing a common definition of what constitutes a profession is far from straightforward or uncontested (Barnett et al 1987, Becher 1999a, Downie 1990). The nature of this debate depends on the critical stance adopted in framing the debate. Downie illustrates this, for example, in examining why the political left would argue that professions are elitist, class biased and profiteering, while the New Right sees them as monopolistic and restrictive. From the perspective of this study, the contested territory is concerned with the nature of knowledge, and the claims of a particular group to have a sufficiently distinctive knowledge to enable them to assert that they work in a way that is different to others and therefore uniquely meets the needs of a client group.

These features are themselves subject to areas of dispute and definitional problems. For example, there are debates around the boundaries between professions and occupations (Etzioni 1969, Rolls 1997), which may be related to either the scope of the knowledge base or the relationship to their customer or client group.

Similarly, there may be a blurring of the definitions around 'minimally competent to practice' and 'fully competent to practice', which implies distinguishing between entry level and expertise or mastery. This can be complex, when individuals are highly competent in some areas but have only a general knowledge in others. Determining the relationship between sub-groupings in terms of their relative competence implies a managerial perspective on professionalism, which may conflict with the normative collegiality inherent in the notion of a single professional body.

Within one profession, it must now be questioned whether identity can be seen as anything other than 'collective specialist activity' (Becher 1999a, p. 83). Similarly, subdisciplines can be conceptualized as minorities within a profession that challenge the notion of one shared sense of professional identity, and explicitly link themselves to groupings outside the professions (Becher 1990). Thus, within a profession, professional identity is neither static nor uncontested. This is particularly true of herbal medicine, with its differing traditions drawn from very different cultural origins.

Downie (1990) argues that there is a complex set of variables around the nature of the service provided for a client when there is also a commercial benefit to the provider. There is an implication within the professional role that the provider of the service may sometimes have to take actions with which the client does not agree. Such actions might suit the wider needs of society rather than the needs of the direct client (as, for example, when an accountant privileges an ethical responsibility to 'true and fair' reporting over the audit report for which clients might believe they are paying). A part of this role may involve speaking out on behalf of society in some area of dispute where the specialist knowledge of professionals renders them competent to espouse an informed view. This expert role implies an independence from financial or political pressure, which will almost certainly manifest itself through the independence and power of the professional body (Giddens 1984).

Such independence and power can vary from one professional body to another. In the case of school teaching, for example, this is expressed as a tension between professionalization and professionalism. This distinction was argued in defence of the proposal to set up a General Teaching Council to make explicit professional values:

"The motive is not to contribute to the process of professionalization, the pursuit of status demands, and all this implies, by which an occupation becomes a profession ... It is to look again at professionalism, the quality of practice, and how members of the profession integrate their obligations with their knowledge and skill in a context of collegiality and contractual and ethical relationships with clients."

(Thompson 1997, p. 5)

So, in making claims to a knowledge and practice that is sufficiently differentiated and substantial to qualify as 'professional' in nature, it is necessary also to consider *who* legitimizes such a claim, as well as *what* is being claimed. It is not sufficient for a group of practitioners to assert that they are a profession; they have to have that claim generally upheld by the public (Glazer 1974). Factors that influence such claims include independence, self-regulation through a professional body, a wider value to society and a distinctive relationship with clients. Conversely, an overly powerful professional body may lose its credibility with the public if it is perceived to retain too much power to itself. It may seem to undervalue the choices, and even the rights, of its clients (as the credibility of the General Medical Council (GMC) can be seen to have been damaged in the early years of this century by a series of mismanaged regulatory cases).

These factors have clear implications for the education of practitioners, as they imply a deep conceptualization of the ways in which professional knowledge may need to be used in practice. The ability to weigh up the real needs of clients as against their own perceived needs, and to manage conflicts between client needs and some wider view of society's needs, suggests a form of professional knowledge that will require discrimination, confidence and ethical judgement. It is likely also to require development over a practitioner's lifetime, as it encompasses a wide mix of skills and knowledge, which will vary with the context of practice. This suggests that a distinctive part of professional identity may reside in the way it approaches education for professional practice. Interestingly, Downie (1990) sees this as one of the more problematic aspects of professional identity:

"Medicine is often taken as the paradigm of a profession, and it does well on all but one of the criteria – being educated as distinct from being trained. Such is the emphasis on the knowledge base and skills that there is a danger that our doctors lack the humane values of the educated mind"

(Downie 1990, p. 155)

This critique is addressed by the GMC (1993), which proposed, among other reforms, a wide range of 'attitudinal objectives' framed around ethical under-standing, an orientation to personal development and the ability to adapt to change.

However, recent research into the implications of the proposed radical reorganizing of initial medical training suggests that the broader aspects of professional education, in particular the 'humanizing' aspect of the curriculum, has only partially changed the nature of provision (Cribb & Bignold 1999). If this is the case with one of the larger and more developed fields, it is evident that a sophisticated understanding of education will be of central importance in the process of establishing a claim to professional status for a new profession. This led to a significant emphasis on education and training in the recommendations of the Herbal Medicine Regulatory Working Group (2003).

When Parliament decided the necessary conditions to allow osteopaths and chiropractors to put themselves forward for recognition and protection of title, they laid emphasis on a number of criteria of the sort we have been discussing, including the need for appropriate professional education. In February 1985, Junior Health Minister Lord Glenarthur introduced five requirements for self-regulation: the profession must be mature, it must have one governing body, it must be based on a systematic body of knowledge, it must have recognized courses of training and it must be able to demonstrate efficacy (Hansard, cited in Copland-Griffiths 1998). These are the tests that are likely to be applied for any other area of complementary medicine that seeks protection of title through statute, as is proposed by acupuncturists as well as herbalists. This collection of essays, examines the implications of attempting to fulfil such requirements.

In summary, the distinctive nature of a profession will be seen to be characterized by:

- a specialist knowledge base, which rests on a framework of ethics
- a relationship of service to clients, which includes some freedom to vary the service delivered in accordance with professional values
- a professional body, which both regulates the ethical conduct of its members and represents its interests to the wider public

- independence from overt external pressure or interference
- broad-based ideas of professional education.

WHO DETERMINES PROFESSIONAL IDENTITY?

If a profession is to have legitimacy in society, it will need to attend to the factors listed above, which give credibility to claims of professional status. Assuming this is done, this next section explores the constituencies with an interest in the recognition of a profession. It discusses the relationship in determining these things between the clients, the practitioners themselves (individually and collectively through their professional body), and the wider public who have a concern for such issues as efficacy and safety. It sets out to map the interest groups who define a profession, and the tensions between the separate interests of these groups.

Earlier professions established themselves by using power structures (Foucault 1980, Johnson 1972). These structures included patronage (which can include communal patronage, dominated by the general public), mediation by the state, and 'true' professionalism, which uses such structural forms as self-regulation and autonomy. Johnson's (1972) account has proved influential in subsequent analyses of professions and professionalization, because of its emphasis on sociocultural factors within the context of the time and place in which a given profession develops. More recently, Thompson (1997) has examined the barriers to developing ideas of the professional status of teachers. She gives equal weight to society's current distrust of professional status, 'a backlash against the power, privileges and pretensions of special interest groups' (p. 4), and to the state's current degree of control:

"Has the State taken so many powers and therefore assumed the right to be the sole determinant of the norms, values and principles which are essential to a teacher's professionalism? "

(Thompson 1997, p.15)

Becher (1999a) reports the results of a large comparative study between the professions of medicine, pharmacy, law, accountancy, architecture and structural engineering. His data suggest that the important variables include the relationships with clients, the impact of professional bodies, the pace of change in the external world (including new legislation and the impact of technology), shifts in status in relationship to other professions and a range of commercial and business factors. For example, he describes how architects have had 'a battering experience' throughout the past decade:

"The interviewees shared the view that they had been deliberately undermined by government policies, and that the quality of their relationships with clients had changed for the worse. They were aware of growing public alienation . . . and [were] stung by the recurrent 'bashing in the press'. "

(Becher 1999a, p. 36)

21

In contrast, Becher suggests that doctors tend to enjoy high social and professional status, but have differentiations within their own internal ranks. Lawyers, in contrast again, seem to have only grudging public respect but high social standing, because of the age of the profession and the hegemony of the professional groupings (p. 28). Within law he discusses, in particular, barristers who remain relatively untouched by some of the determinants of professional identity that operate on their near relations, the solicitors:

"they function as single practitioners, remain staunchly independent and individualistic, actively retain their rituals and traditions and are resistant to attempts to bring them more into keeping with contemporary values and practices."

(Becher 1999a, p. 29)

The fact that, in Becher's research (1999a), no single model of determining professional identity predominates suggests that complex variables are at play in the formation and acceptance of professional status, and that these are not necessarily based on rational criteria. Professional identity can be seen to be a battleground between a number of competing interest groups. These can include sponsors (e.g. professions, governments, employers), providers of education and clients (Churchman & Woodhouse 1999). So the contested nature of professional identity arises, in part, from tensions within and outside the profession.

Within a profession, there can be distinctive subgroupings that act against the interests of the wider group. This may well be attributable to what Becher (1990) has designated as the 'counterculture of specialization'. The claims of new knowledge, and interdisciplinary working, can lead to fragmentation within a profession, to new professional groupings; more positively, they can help to develop a shared sense of purpose in terms of special interest groups (such as the Royal Colleges in medicine). In herbal medicine, some of these tensions have arisen within traditions from very different cultural origins.

In particular, the position of professional members within educational settings can raise some interesting tensions (Eraut 1994, Rolls 1997). Such individuals may feel torn between the different cultures, purposes and values of professional and academic life. At the level of initial training, such tensions can lead to the creation of 'an alienating education', where the necessary socialization of an incomer into professional life is perceived as in conflict with the desirable encouragement of an active and critical engagement with the discourse of the profession (Burwood 1999). Alternatively, newcomers into a profession may encounter an oppositional approach in their first educators, which has its roots in an adherence to the idea of a university as in some sense apart from society, with a critical stance to the instrumentalism of initial education (Kogan 1999).

Thus we see that the stakeholders who determine professional identity include:

- the state, and policy makers
- the general public, including patients
- the professional body
- interest groups of practitioners
- the higher education community.

HOW ARE THE DETERMINANTS OF PROFESSIONAL IDENTITY MANIFESTED?

There are a variety of means by which the above stakeholders can influence the way professional identity is determined. As we have seen, this can start with the socialization of the new beginner into the profession, at the point of initial training. This can work to discourage the active participation of students in forming their personal understandings of the meaning of professional identity, because of a desire to transmit the generic style of the discipline (Burwood 1999). Alternatively, students can be insufficiently prepared for the networks of relationships that come with professional identity because of the 'aloof' setting of a university (Eraut et al 1995). Less usually, but of importance to this study, the practitioner community can dominate the socialization process by having primary responsibility for the education of new entrants, through colleges outside the mainstream education sector. These may suffer from reluctance to develop new professional knowledge or unwillingness to deviate significantly from occupational regulations (Eraut 1994, p. 6).

As individuals' own careers progress through differing contexts, they will encounter in each context an embedding of a different social construction of practice. Eraut (2000) suggests that such individuals develop personal variations from professional norms through such experiences. It is interesting to ask whether such individual changes might, over time, aggregate to change the professional body norms, or whether they remain private and personal (Giddens 1991a).

More structural ways of determining professional identity are the methods of controlling entry to the profession through less formal gate-keeping processes or more formal accreditation systems (Becher 1999b, Churchman & Woodhouse 1999). These regulatory processes can be extended to systems for continuous education, including compulsory reregistration at intervals (Becher 1999a). As a corollary to these, there may be restrictions on the use of particular titles. Such control mechanisms can originate in the opposition of more powerful professions to subgroupings or specialisms that seek professional recognition in their own right (Melville 1998). Structural controls encompass a range of methods, including statutory regulation, statutory self-regulation, protection of title and voluntary regulation.

The mechanisms that regulate professional identity and behaviour, and influence perceptions of its standing and credibility, include:

- socialization into professional mores
- course accreditation
- requirements for professional updating or relicensing
- regulation
- protection of title.

All of these issues are addressed in the report of the Herbal Medicine Regulatory Working Group (2003).

It is worth noting here that the interest group that seems to have the least influence on the ways in which professions develop is the client or patient group. In part, this can be seen to be a reflection of the fragmented nature of such a population. There is also an inequality of power between the ability of practitioners to operate collectively and the individualized identity of clients. However, the relative lack of influence of patients also may result from unwillingness on the part of practitioners to recognize the generalizability of individual patient experiences in the context of generating a critical understanding of the service ethic in practice:

*"Interestingly, whereas there is typically little questioning of the nature and legitimacy of the representatives of **educators** or speakers from **professional practice**, the perceived 'failure' of users to be representative can be hotly debated by students [of social work] and there may be intense discussion about accepting the views of lay people who do not meet some quite often unspecified criteria for representativeness."*

(Taylor 1997, p.178; my emphasis)

The Herbal Medicine Regulatory Working Group addressed this by the inclusion of lay members representing the patient interest among its members. The issues relating to the patient interest are discussed by Michael Pittilo in the third section of this volume.

In this section, we have discussed some of the influences that lead to the formation of professions. One of these is the desire of practitioners to come together to improve knowledge. A second reason is their suppression of internal dissent in the interests of regulation and protection of title where they are threatened by the possibility of others practising their skill. The impact of all these divergent influences and interest groups is to impose some form of overall coherence on a group of disparate professionals, so that they can come together and say 'we are a profession'.

This cohesion may happen differently at different times, representing the dynamic nature of professions. Taylor (1997, p. 17, adapting Abrams & Bulmer) describes four types of relationships between interest groups. These are:

- *colonization*, where one group invades or subordinates another, either by dominating their agenda or by appropriating their role
- *conflict*, which may result from this, and represents an explicit response to the colonizer from those within the profession
- *confusion*, which may or may not be a response to colonization, and manifests itself in conflicting discourses and values; it can be seen as a positive experience where there is explicit acknowledgement and discussion of multiple perspectives
- *integration*, which is the stage where there is power sharing in the interest of value creation.

In the earliest days of a new profession, the recently established professional body may feel colonized by ideas from outside about its ethics and professional practices, and it may not be allowed to exist without putting certain processes in place (such as published minimum standards for entry into practice). As the profession struggles to come to terms with these requirements, it is likely to experience both conflict and confusion, as it seeks to understand the impact of change on its own internal understandings of professional identity and professional knowledge. As it becomes established, gains general recognition and starts to feel more powerful, the profession is more likely to be able to use ideas from the wider community to continue to develop its knowledge base. This last stage represents integration, and may well manifest itself through the exercise of choice over the management of tensions between the concepts of knowledge, service to clients and professional autonomy.

IN WHAT WAYS DO PROFESSIONS DIFFER FROM ONE ANOTHER?

So far, we have considered some of the common characteristics of professions, and the ways that external threats to these characteristics can act as agents for movement towards homogeneity among diverse groups within a profession.

This sort of process is by no means a linear one, and professions differ with the speed at which they change, the solutions they find to some of the problems of professionalism, and the relative weight they attach to different aspects of professional knowledge. These differences and distinctions are compounded by the recent tendency of professions to work together cooperatively in delivering services to clients. Increasingly, such cooperation extends to the foundation of common principles of education, to the point sometimes of sharing core modules:

"By these means, professions formed alliances to enhance their status in relation to one another and the more established professions, notably medicine."

(Barr et al 1999, p. 535)

In order, however, to establish the ways in which herbalism and acupuncture can be considered distinctive as professions, it is necessary to explore some of the ways in which professions differ. This will allow for some discussion of the choices (implicit and explicit) that can shape professional development and education.

The distinctions cited by Eraut (1994) at the start of this chapter can be used as a framework to discuss this question. The first of his categories is a specialist knowledge base. Different professions have different ideas about the nature of a knowledge base that might be appropriate for professional practice, as is illustrated by Barnett et al (1987) in their comparison of initial professional education in pharmacy, nursing and teacher education. This study remains one of the most distinctive discussions of alternative approaches to professional knowledge in the literature. However, their study, having been carried out in the late 1980s, does not distinguish between contrasting conceptualizations of different kinds of professional knowledge in action (using concepts developed by Schon 1987, Eraut 1994 and later commentators).

Barnett et al (1987) suggest that differences in the ways professions define their knowledge base are derived from a number of different causes. The first of these is the orientation of the discipline towards the sciences or the humanities. The second is the relationship between theory and practice. A third difference is the extent to which initial training relies on learning through doing. Finally, a fourth dimension relates to the research activity of the community. These distinctions, epistemological and pedagogical, are examined further in Section Three by Nick Lampert (Chapter 10) and Alison Denham (Chapter 11).

The second characteristic of professions is autonomy of practice (Barnett et al 1987, Eraut 1994). For many professional groups this has changed considerably from the settings in which practitioners worked in the early days of professionalism. It has been argued that a key factor influencing professional autonomy is the professional body structures. The stronger the professional body's grip on the curriculum the greater is the independence of the profession (Barnett et al 1987). Related to this is the relationship between the practitioner community and the academic group who take responsibility for preparation for practice. The stronger these links, the more appropriate is the preparation for the professional context.

Thirdly, the service ideal and the way it is conceptualized can be a defining difference between professions (Eraut 1994, Thompson 1997). Different professions have different ideas about the relative importance of service users and service purchasers, and about the reciprocal nature of interactions with clients. In education terms, this has important implications for the timing of the introduction of students to the ambiguities of clinical reality or the practice setting. Where some part of the training consists of gaining practical experience in the workplace, there are implications for the expectations made of students when they encounter clients at different points in their training (Eraut et al 1995, Taylor 1997). The complexities of the context of service delivery can vary greatly between professions, as may be illustrated by comparing the roles of a GP and a community pharmacist. Such distinctions lead to important questions concerning the relationship between initial training and continuous professional development, the orientation of learners towards their own development and the structures that deliver such learning most effectively.

So, some of the ways in which a new profession can develop for itself a conceptualization of what is meant by professionalism through educational processes is by developing a clear perspective on the following:

- the theoretical knowledge of the profession
- the relationship between theory and practice
- the extent that initial learning includes practice experience
- the ways new knowledge is constructed
- the orientation of individuals to their own development
- the role of the professional body in education
- the relationship between professional knowledge and other forms of knowledge (arts/humanities/sciences)
- the status of the profession vis-à-vis other professions and the higher education community.

THE RELATIONSHIPS BETWEEN PROFESSIONS AND HIGHER EDUCATION IN TERMS OF KNOWLEDGE

So far we have examined the ideas of professions as idealized social and cultural phenomena. We have looked at some of the forces that determine professional identity, and at some of the mechanisms different professions use to render themselves distinct and to position themselves relative to others. We have seen that professional identity is contested, and that it is greatly influenced by forces external to it and therefore largely outside its direct control. Thus a profession interacts dynamically with its context (Becher 1999a), and seeks to influence and control external pressures by decisions made over professional values, service delivery and the knowledge base.

There is thus an inherent tension in the way that a profession views knowledge. This tension resides in the difference between viewing knowledge as a way of defining professional legitimacy and viewing it as a means of improving the service offered to clients. In other words, there is a tension between the normative and the instrumental view of knowledge creation.

Historically, knowledge has been deemed to be the province of higher education (Barnett 1994, Boyer 1990). Within higher education, however, there are very distinctive differences observable between disciplines (Becher 1994, Eljamal et al 1999). Becher (1999a, preface) observes that the professionally orientated subject areas seem harder to characterize than their 'pure' counterparts. Some of the possible reasons for this have already been discussed in the above exploration of the problematic nature of professions, and therefore of professional education.

Professional knowledge can be viewed as problematic because it is closely allied to, and often confused with, issues around the power and status of professions, particularly with regard to the respect offered by the public to practitioners and the financial rewards to be earned from professional services. There is an inherent tension between the profession itself (with a personal stake in the outcome) and the higher education community. This tension resides in the expectation of the higher education community about who legitimizes the claims of the knowledge base.

Disciplinary differences arise in part from epistemological concerns and in part from social and cultural ones. Epistemology, in particular, has hitherto been uniquely the province of higher education (Barnett 1994). Within higher education, there is a hierarchy of rigour, and also an underacknowledged susceptibility to fashion (Becher 1990). This means that within the higher education community itself there are very different ideas about what constitutes acceptable knowledge. This may be particularly problematic where the knowledge in question is derived from non-Western cultures, but is also the case for traditional forms of Western medicine that challenge the orthodox model.

The notion that universities are the place where knowledge claims are validated, and disciplinary groupings are legitimized, is itself under challenge (Brew 1999, Johnston 1998). Forces within the university sector are, to some extent, working against the culture of new knowledge creation (McNeill 1999). This resistance can arise from policies of the state such as inspections of teaching and research, or internal pressures such as contracts and organizational structures. The role of the university in knowledge creation and knowledge generation is increasingly contested at a macro level (Barnett 1994). This same process can be seen at departmental level, with potential tensions between the organizational structures and the natural academic groupings of different disciplines.

Becher (1994, p. 152) compares two ways of categorizing what he calls 'intellectual clusters', drawing on the work of Biglan (1973) and Kolb (1981). This suggests that different disciplines orientate themselves differently in terms of their epistemologies and cognitive processes. From this analysis, Becher (1994) derives a taxonomy of disciplinary groupings, which maps attitudes to knowledge against cultural characteristics. At the macro level, such an analysis has proved problematic for herbal medicine as a discrete discipline, because it spans the range of factors identified by Becher (1994) as significant. Herbal medicine shares the holistic concerns Becher associates with the humanities, has the pragmatic concerns he identifies with a 'hard-applied' discipline, and the uncertainties of status he associates with the 'soft-applied' areas such as teaching. The difficulties in fitting herbal medicine into this model both illustrates the ways in which it is culturally and epistemologically distinct (perhaps because of its Eastern origins in the case of the Chinese, Tibetan and Ayurveda systems) and at the same time confirms the emphasis Becher (1994) puts on cultural factors in influencing disciplinary differences.

Within the higher education community, ideas of knowledge creation are bound up with ideas of academic rigour, institutional pressures, and an array of factors around prestige and career development. The same tensions can be observed in the ways professions seek to locate themselves in terms of their epistemology. The nature of the knowledge base is inextricably linked to questions of autonomy and status. The practice of medicine is a 'hard-applied' science, whereas that of nursing or psychotherapy is a 'soft-applied' one (using Biglan's 1973 descriptors, cited by Becher 1994). However, doctors enjoy very different freedoms to nurses to practice autonomously, and are given much greater status in society with all that brings with it in terms of money and prestige. Therefore, behind the questions around the evidence base for professional claims to knowledge, there lies an unresolved issue about the place of a new profession in society, and the way this is shaped according to the value society places on different sorts of knowledge.

Thus there exist two distinct groups, both of whom have a stake in the creation and validation of knowledge, and both of whom experience tensions around the prestige and status of different kinds of knowledge. Inevitably therefore, when these two groups come together, there will be potential conflict over control of the professional knowledge base, and the responsibility for inducting new entrants into the profession. Issues of differential power will inevitably arise, with those who have power seeking to protect and retain it, while those who lack it try to gain it through alliances and power broking.

Barnett (1994) argues, in effect, that society as a whole is increasingly disinclined to leave knowledge creation to special interest groups that may subordinate knowledge to self-serving ends:

"Crudely speaking, society is coming to determine the forms of knowing that it wishes for itself."

(Barnett 1994, p. 22)

He suggests a number of causes for this. The first of these is an overreliance on cognition within academic communities, and a consequent undervaluing of the sorts of knowledge widely used in ordinary life (Atkinson & Claxton 2000). A second reason is globalization and, related to that, the development of the knowledge society (Giddens 1991b). To Barnett's analysis, we can add the loss of faith in professionals that has been discussed earlier in this chapter (academics occupy a professional place in society, although they do not fulfil some of the characteristics of professionals discussed earlier). In addition there is a more general loss of faith in expertise, in the wake of such incidents as the BSE outbreak or the attempt to introduce genetically modified crops for reasons that the public clearly found insufficiently transparent. This could be construed as representing a certain dissonance between the values placed on certain kinds of knowledge by service users and by those who shape policy (Delanty 2001).

Barnett (1994, p. 172ff.) further argues that some of the dissatisfactions of wider society with the narrower views of knowledge in universities are to do with the mind/body dualism of Western thought. This results in a separation of cognitive knowledge from other ways of knowing, which is related to a Cartesian emphasis on reason (Atkinson & Claxton 2000). Barnett suggests, without actually using these words, that this narrower view of knowledge does not match the zeitgeist, and offers an alternative way of conceptualizing knowledge, which he calls 'lifeworld becoming' (Habermas 1978). This sort of a conception of knowledge, which combines and integrates operational and academic competence, seems particularly suited to professional knowledge and particularly to those professions that work holistically. This may in part explain the greater willingness of some universities to offer programmes in herbal medicine.

Thus, in summary, there are contested areas around who determines knowledge. Hitherto, there has been a hierarchy of knowledge, which privileges some forms as being more important than others. This means that it is important to a profession to be linked to the 'right' form of knowledge in terms of status. Higher education ideas of 'right' form may not agree with other groups (e.g. the general public). A new profession has to manage the tensions of the interrelationships between itself and the higher education community, itself and society, and itself and its knowledge base. Given this level of complexity, this is likely to result in considerable fluidity, conflict and change. The third section of this study explores a number of different ways in which such fluidity, conflict and changes were experienced within the different communities of herbal medicine at a particular historical moment.

CONCLUSION

In this chapter, we have looked at a number of ways in which professional identity can be determined, challenged and evolved. We considered the nature of professions, and their defining characteristics, which revolve around specialist knowledge, a distinctive service and professional autonomy. These are underpinned by broad concepts of values, ethics and adaptability. The next part of the chapter examined further the constituencies who have a stake in the development and legitimization of professional identity. These include subgroupings inside and outside the profession, and the interests of these groups will inevitably sometimes come into conflict. The resolution of such conflict often depends on the perceived power of the profession. Education plays a significant part in establishing the credibility of a profession in the eyes of society. At the same time, it is in the spaces opened up by education that some of the tensions between knowledge as science and knowledge as culture are played out (Delanty 2001).

The significance of the theory in relation to herbal medicine lies in the depiction of complexity in relation to professional identity. We have seen that professional identity is neither static nor uncontested. Some commentators argue that it is the changes in the external context that impact on changing conceptualizations of professionalism. Others lay greater emphasis on internal influences, identifying a range of factors about which choices can be made. Clearly power and special interest groups have a part to play in this. Furthermore, the relative power of the professional body is of significance in questions of status and independence. These are therefore the areas of influence that this study will need to investigate in order to establish the drivers for change in the development of professionalism in herbal medicine.

Knowledge and educational processes too are complex and problematic areas for professions. The next chapter will look in more detail at issues in professional education, focusing the discussion in terms of the impact of education on the socialization of the individual into an extended conceptualization of professional identity.

References

Atkinson T, Claxton G 2000 The intuitive practitioner. Open University Press, Buckingham

Barnett R 1994 The limits of competence: knowledge, higher education and society. Society for Research into Higher Education/Open University Press, Buckingham.

Barnett R, Becher T, Cork N 1987 Models of professional preparation: Pharmacy, Nursing and Teacher Education. Studies in Higher Education 12(1):51–63

Barr H, Hammick M, Koppell I et al 1999 Evaluating inter-professional education: two systematic reviews for health and social care. British Education Research Journal 25(4):530–535

Becher T 1990 The counter-culture of specialisation. European Journal of Education 25(3):333–347

Becher T 1994 The significance of disciplinary differences. Studies in Higher Education 19(2):151–161

Becher T 1999a Professional practices: commitment and capability in a changing environment. Transaction, New Brunswick

Becher T 1999b Quality in the professions. Studies in Higher Education 24(2):225–235

Biglan A 1973 The characteristics of subject matter in different scientific areas. Journal Of Applied Psychology 57:195–203

Boyer E L 1990 Scholarship reconsidered: priorities of the professoriate. Carnegie Foundation, Princeton NJ

Brew A 1999 Research and teaching: changing relationships in a changing context. Studies in Higher Education 24(3):291–301

Burwood S 1999 Liberation philosophy. Teaching in Higher Education 4(4):447–460

Churchman R, Woodhouse D 1999 The influence of professional and statutory bodies on professional schools within New Zealand tertiary institutions. Quality in Higher Education 5(3):211–226

Copland-Griffiths M C 1998 Statutory regulation – the chiropractic experience. European Journal of Oriental Medicine 2(6):4–11

Cribb A, Bignold S 1999 Towards a reflexive medical school: the hidden curriculum and medical education research. Studies in Higher Education 24(2):195–209

Delanty G 2001 Challenging knowledge: the university in the knowledge society. Open University Press, Buckingham

Downie R S 1990 Professions and professionalism. Journal of the Philosophy of Education 24(2):147–159

Eljamal M B, Stark J S, Arnold G L et al 1999 Intellectual development: a complex teaching goal. Studies in Higher Education 24(1):15–25

Eraut M 1994 Developing professional knowledge and competence. Falmer, London

Eraut M 2000 Non-formal learning and tacit knowledge in professional work. British Journal of Educational Psychology 70:113–136

Eraut M, Alderton J, Boylan A et al 1995 Learning to use scientific knowledge in education and practicum settings: an evaluation of the contribution of the biological, behavioural and social sciences to pre-registration nursing and midwifery courses. English National Board for Nursing, Midwifery and Health Visiting, London

Etzioni A 1969 The semi-professions and their organisation, Free Press, New York

Foucault, M 1980 Power/knowledge; selected interviews and other writings. Pantheon, New York

General Medical Council 1993 Tomorrow's doctors: recommendations on undergraduate medical education. General Medical Council, London

Giddens A 1984 The constitution of society: outline of the theory of structuration. Polity Press, Cambridge

Giddens A 1991a The consequences of modernity. Polity Press, Cambridge

Giddens A 1991b Modernity and self-identity: self and society in the late Modern Age. Polity Press, Cambridge

Glazer N 1974 The schools of the minor professions. Minerva 12(3):346–363

Habermas J 1978 Knowledge and human interest. Heinemann, London

Herbal Medicine Regulatory Working Group 2003 Recommendations on the regulation of herbal practitioners. Prince of Wales's Foundation for Integrated Health, London

Johnson 1972 Professions and power. Macmillan, London

Johnston R 1998 The university of the future: Boyer revisited. Higher Education 36:253–272

Kogan M 1999 Higher education communities and academic identity. Paper presented at the Society for Research into Higher Education, UMIST

Kolb D A 1981 Learning styles and disciplinary differences. In: Chickering A (ed) The modern American college. Jossey Bass, San Francisco, pp 231–255

McIntyre D 1994 Preface. In Eraut (1994) Developing professional knowledge and competence. Falmer, London

McNeill D 1999 On inter-disciplinary research: with particular reference to the field of environment and development. Higher Education Quarterly 53(4):312–332

Melville E 1998 Statutory regulation – no easy answers. European Journal of Oriental Medicine 2(6):51–54

Rolls E 1997 Competence in professional practice: some issues and concerns.
    Educational Research 32(2):195–210

Schon D A 1987 Educating the reflective practitioner. Jossey-Bass, San Francisco

Taylor I 1997 Developing learning in professional education; partnerships for practice.
    Society for Research into Higher Education/Open University Press, Buckingham

Thompson M 1997 Professional ethics and the teacher: towards a General Teaching
    Council. Trentham Books, Stoke on Trent

Whitty D 1999 Teacher professionalism and the state in the 21st century. Paper
    presented at the Standing Committee for the Education and Training of Teachers,
    Dunchurch, Rugby

Professional education and practitioner identity

2

Catherine O'Sullivan

OVERVIEW

In the preceding chapter, which looked at the macro organization of professions, it has been argued that education is one of the critical variables in determining the status of professions. This chapter is concerned with professional education, with specific relationship to the micro level of the development of an individual practitioner for the context of professional practice. It relates to the detailed recommendations made on the entry-level curriculum, accreditation and continuous professional development in the report of the Herbal Medicine Regulatory Working Group (2003).

The chapter discusses the relationship between the practitioner's own values and personal knowing, their capability for practice, and the generation of a more abstract evidence base. It is suggested that it is in the ways that groups of individual practitioners collectively build shared understandings of such relationships that professional identity is forged.

THE NATURE OF KNOWLEDGE FOR PROFESSIONAL PRACTICE

The initial distinction between professional education and other forms of higher education was focused on the relationship between *knowing how* and *knowing that* (Dreyfus & Dreyfus 1986, Kolb 1984, Ryle 1949). This was developed by Eraut (1994) into a distinction between three kinds of knowing: propositional, process and personal knowledge. Each of these has been sub-divided, as we shall see, into disparate classifications that seek to typify the subtleties of the kinds of knowledge that need to be drawn on in the multiplicities of ways that knowledge is applied in the context of practice.

Allied to this discussion of the types of knowledge used in professional practice is a related discussion about the ways such knowledge is accessed and used. This relates to ideas about conscious and unconscious decision making, tacit knowledge and implicit and explicit modes of cognition. These debates about the ways knowledge is used in practice inevitably spawned a related interest in how such knowledge can be acquired in relation to a practitioner's learning and to strategies for the teaching of professionals.

A different school of thought has concentrated less on the *how* of learning and looked more at the *where*. This approach emphasizes the specificity of the context for learning and argues that, as all knowledge is socially and culturally constructed, it can be learnt only through a gradual socialization into the community of practitioners. This socialization is based on learning through doing, supported by a dialogue with more senior colleagues (Lave & Wenger 1991). By taking a holistic approach to learning, adherents of this school avoid the necessity to draw ever-closer distinctions between types of knowledge and their application in practice. It does, however, beg the question of how individuals learn who are largely separate from a community (i.e. those professionals who practise in the context of autonomy). This will prove to be a problematic area in the context of the statutory self-regulation of herbal practitioners.

A strength of the Lave & Wenger (1991) model of professional education is its emphasis on the 'legitimate' and the 'peripheral' ways that beginners become full members of the community of practice. This acknowledges both the gradual and evolutionary way that professional knowledge is acquired and refined and also the stake that the rest of the profession has in the formation of professional expertise. An important dimension to professional learning is the relationship between initial training and continuous professional development, whether or not this is formally prescribed and regulated. Probably the most influential model for this development is the five-stage process developed by Dreyfus & Dreyfus (1986). This describes the stages through which a practitioner passes as novice, advanced beginner, competent, proficient and expert. The model shows the gradual replacement of a reliance on rules and overt procedures as the ability to form rapid, intuitive judgements of the whole situation develops.

Thus, in the field of professional education, there a number of factors that need to be considered, which are interrelated. The first of these are the forms of professional knowledge. The second is the way knowledge is used in practice. The third involves the way that individuals acquire knowledge. It is then important to consider how this is supported through professional life, past the early stages of development. Finally, it is necessary to look at teaching and learning, and strategies for developing research, in the context of individuals within a larger community of professionals.

HOW DO INDIVIDUALS LEARN THEIR PROFESSION?

The context of knowledge acquisition

Historically, most professions began to teach their trade to new entrants by a system of apprenticeship or pupillage. This involves the learner being bound to the master, usually for a defined period of time. Learners offer their services to the master at a cheap price and, in exchange, they learn their trade and pass into full membership of their profession. The remnants of this system can still be seen in the way, for example, barristers gain admittance to the bar. It is a particularly powerful model for herbal medicine, as it is still the way that practitioners learn in some parts of India, Sri Lanka, China and Tibet.

Here in the UK, it has tended to be superseded by the formation of institutions whose main purpose is the preparation of practitioners (such as the Central School of Speech and Drama), or by the establishment of specific programmes within larger educational institutions, most usually universities. Some professions may have statutory pressure to make such a transition, as in the recent cases of teaching and nursing:

"the British government's current attempts to remove initial teacher education from the higher education sector contrast not only with the French government's radical moves in the opposite direction but also with the British government's own support for the movement of initial nurse education into higher education"

(author's emphasis; McIntyre 1994, p. ix)

At the time of this publication, the professions of herbal medicine can be seen to be in transition between these states, with some education delivered within specialist colleges and others being trained in universities. A considerable number of individuals still learn herbal medicine by studying alongside another member of the profession, and the differences in quality of these experiences is part of the background to the professional accreditation processes.

In their study of nurse education, Eraut et al (1995) discuss some of the implications of the move into higher education. They suggest that it can lead to the codification of large areas of professional knowledge into textbooks, which are not useful in teaching students about the application of technical knowledge in practice. The value to them of the higher education model lies in the internationally recognized currency of awards, the general education that is delivered in universities and the independence of universities in the creation and validation of knowledge (p. 36). However, they feel this move can also lead to a split between theory and practice, and a devaluing of practical expertise as such knowledge is not valued as highly as academic knowledge.

In their study of the initial training of nurses and midwives in seven institutional settings, they conclude that the quality of the educational processes offered is, in many cases, quite inappropriate to the needs of students. The factors they identify include:

- the need to mediate theory in practice settings
- the timing of the introduction of theory in terms of the student's development in clinical knowledge
- the need for good mentoring or coaching in the practice settings
- the impact of the students' socialization into the profession.

This last point is particularly interesting because they find:

"There is always tension between leading professionals, who aspire to raise their profession's status and standards of practice by increasing use of scientific knowledge, and ordinary practitioners whose defensive responses stem from their wish to do the job they have always known ... Many students rationalised their limited knowledge by claiming that 'good' practitioners did not appear to need it ..."

(Eraut et al 1995, p. 99)

Their work suggests that professional socialization can be a force that either supports or inhibits the development of students, depending on the practice context in which students are working. The move into higher education of initial training can alter the dynamic of this socialization process, causing a tension between academic and practicum teachers, which may also be influenced by the attitude of the professional body towards initial training.

This conclusion is borne out by another study that looked at learning across seven professions: 'The view that their professional bodies were remote and out of touch with what was going on was expressed by quite a few individuals in most professions' (Gear et al 1994, p. 57). This resulted in a reduction in the influence of the profession on the way new practitioners acquired knowledge appropriate for practice.

However, this same study found that informal contact between professionals was valued by practitioners in terms of direct learning, and with the valued-added benefits of building relationships, trust and new networks. A consequent danger was acknowledged if the pool of fellow professionals was too limited, 'It was pointed out that it could be unhelpful, even dangerous, if bad habits or practices were picked up' (Gear et al 1994, p. 31).

Both these studies covered quite large samples. Gear's involved 150 participants and Eraut et al interviewed and observed 187 people in a variety of settings and activities. They thus offer good empirical evidence of the problems with programmes of professional learning at the point at which they relate to individual learners. A third study, conducted by Eraut et al (1998), looked at how individuals from three professions learnt at work, and covered a sample of 120 people from business, engineering and healthcare. These studies represent a major addition to the evidence base of professional education, centred on the experiences of practitioners. They exposed some dissonance between the explicit aims of educators and professional bodies, and the impact on the learning of the individual.

The relationship between initial training and continuous professional development

Gear et al (1994), Eraut et al (1995) and Eraut et al (1998) all consider the relationship between initial training and continuous professional development (CPD). In particular, they raise questions about the ways in which early experiences in professional life may have a beneficial or an adverse impact on the propensity of the individual to continue to learn into their future life.

"The inadequacy of initial professional education as a preparation for one's entire working life is now well recognised by professional bodies ... The picture that emerges finally from this study is of an activity which is primarily initiated, organised, resourced and evaluated by individuals and their colleagues. Indeed, it is difficult to see how anything else could be consistent with the notion of a profession ..."

(Gear et al 1994, p. 79)

Although this statement suggests that it is a characteristic of professionals to be in control of their own learning, it does not consider that this autonomy is in itself a skill that needs to be acquired during the initial training. Particularly for those professions who recruit students straight from school, a concern for their own developmental needs is something to be fostered in the early years of education and practice.

From the perspective of the professional body, this can be an issue that needs to be held in dynamic tension:

"We found that formal education and training contribute to only a small proportion of learning at work ... the most frequently discussed issues in initial training for the professions concern (1) the need for breadth or specialization and (2) the balance and phasing of learning and education in workplace contexts"

(Eraut et al 1998, p. 19)

This tension can be fuelled by external bodies with an interest in the raising of standards. This gives the professional body the role of both withstanding this pressure and providing for postregistration activities and needs:

"as the knowledge base grows, increased pressure is put on the pre-registration curriculum ... but [registration] should never be regarded as a summit of professional learning. It is more appropriate to consider a series of transitions, continuing across the point of registration, in which greater responsibility is gradually assumed and the range of duties is widened."

(Eraut et al 1995, p.105)

Thus recent research evidence seems to suggest that learners learn best from gradual exposure to practice, and that it is not effective to front-load the curriculum, particularly with technical knowledge that does not make sense until it is experienced within the realities of the work context. The impact of others in the workplace is of great importance in this developing learning:

"Much professional knowledge seems to be relatively unsystematic, subtle and tacit ... This emphasis on the importance of contact between both experts and novices and among peers tallies with some of the more recent research on the nature of professional expertise, in terms of the

*importance placed on 'modelling' and what might be called embedded
and embodied learning ..."*

(Gear et al 1994, p. 76)

So, a tension is being set up between, on the one hand, the desire of the professional bodies to ensure entry levels into the profession are of a high standard and, on the other hand, the inability of the individual learner to make sense of learning outside the professional context in which it is practised. This latter difficulty also includes the inability to make sense of the whole picture, rather than of the separate pieces of theory that together impact on a situation in practice. Many workplace problems will involve utilizing multiple theories in an integrated way, and prioritizing the relative importance of the different elements. These sorts of judgements are difficult to learn outside the practice setting:

*"students were unused to activities which systematically studied the
knowledge base relevant to a particular case"*

(Eraut et al 1995, p. 115).

Thus, it can be argued, the initial training curriculum should be developing the study skills to make sense of complex situations, where a range of sorts of knowledge are needed. CPD can then be used to inform these judgements with more sophisticated technical material, when the student is sufficiently competent to apply it with discrimination.

Types of knowledge for professional practice

Elsewhere in the same study (Eraut et al 1995, p. 13), the authors conclude that there are four types of process knowledge involved in professional learning:

- acquiring and interpreting information about clients and situations
- deciding how to respond in the short and longer term
- implementing actions
- meta processes including directing and controlling their own behaviour and ongoing monitoring of clients and their environment.

A curriculum for professional education has to consider these types of process knowledge. A novice practitioner gains experience and develops process knowledge, which utilizes propositional knowledge within the practicum setting. Alongside this, the individual needs mechanisms to facilitate the integration of this learning with the considerable stock of prior knowledge that has been gained from life experiences prior to entry into the profession. The unification and integration of different kinds of knowledge and learning can be described as the creation of a competent practitioner (Chapter 11).

The most recent work in the area of professional education suggests that much of this personal knowledge is relatively inaccessible to the practitioner

(Eraut 2000). The current emphasis on the development of the reflective practitioner represents an effort by professional educators to enable practitioners
to access their learning, and to modify it, more easily.

"Reflective practitioners need to develop a critical understanding of
service settings, their historical evolution and current culture to
appreciate the problems and possibilities of change and the tensions that
can arise when changes in practice are proposed. They also need to
understand the extent to which observed and alternative forms of
practice are supported by research and scientific knowledge."

(Eraut et al 1995, p. 112)

The idea of the reflective practitioner incorporates not just complex ideas
about the types of knowledge that are used in professional practice, but also
the ways in which individual practitioners can access this knowledge. This is
based on developments in psychological understandings of the ways knowledge
can be utilized in different practice situations, depending on typologies of tacit
knowledge in use (Eraut 2000). These understandings are new and relatively
undertheorized, but suggest that a greater understanding of the relationship
between professional decision-making processes and modes of cognition will
allow for improvements in professional education.

As this field develops, it is influencing the theoretical understanding of the
ways in which the development of 'the reflective practitioner' relates to the
ways professionals use tacit and intuitive knowledge in a variety of contexts.
Increasingly, for the practitioner, an understanding of the range of strategies
employed, and the sorts of knowledge that are being utilized, will (it is argued)
lead to greater professional discrimination and judgement.

Key influences on the development of reflection

Reflection and reflective practice as techniques in the education of the
professional originated, in the form in which it tends to be understood today,
with Schon (1987), following earlier work (Argyris & Schon 1974). These ideas
were then developed to model ways in which reflective practice can be used to
develop professional ways of knowing. For example, Johns (1995) married
Schon's work to Carper's earlier (1978) framework to emphasize the multidimensional aspects of professional practice. The value of this approach resides
in particular in the weight given to forms of knowledge other than the
technical or skills-based kind (i.e. her emphasis on the artistry of practice, and
of personal knowledge and aesthetic (or ethical) awareness).

Schon's work, being so influential in the development of professional
education, still merits critical attention. He raises important questions about
the nature of professional knowledge, the relationship between theory and
practice, that between professionals in action and professional educators and
the important issue of the role of coaching in the transmission of professional

expertise. This latter point has interesting implications for a field whose early training borrowed the Chinese or Indian model of long apprenticeship to a master whose expertise should not be openly questioned. The purposeful dialogue between coach and learner discussed by Schon (1987) is a long way from this, but it would be easy for his work to be misinterpreted within the particular traditions of herbal medicine education.

Eraut (1995) offers a sympathetic development of Schon's work that, while recognizing some of its inconsistencies, still sees his work as of central importance in developing what Eraut calls a metacognition of professional education. This interest in the metacognition of professionals is developed in Eraut's later work (Eraut et al 1998), and has led to the development of a number of typologies of non-formal learning, tacit knowledge and professional performance (Eraut 2000). This latter work represents a theoretical analysis of the issues and phenomena to do with the ways professionals work, based on the empirical studies Eraut and his colleagues were carrying out through the 1990s. It thus unites theoretical understandings of modes of cognition with theories of professional decision making, and considers both as phenomena that can be individually or socially constructed.

For groupings of professionals who tend to work in conditions of autonomy (e.g. barristers, community pharmacists and those practitioners who are the focus of this present study), there are difficulties in the idea of professional education as a social activity located in the context of 'the learning organization'. Although such professional groups will have extended peer networks, most of their practice activity, with its consequential opportunities for learning and developing tacit theories of practice, happens alone. This suggests an even greater importance for personal knowledge and subjective experience for such professionals. It also raises an interesting question about the rigour of such knowledge, if it is not offered to a peer group for critical appraisal. It has implications for the pace of professional development and the transmission of good practice throughout the community of practitioners.

Reflection can be construed as a link between new learners and the CPD of practitioners. It can serve as a bridge between the personal theories of individuals and more public evidence of good practice. However, there is a shortage of published, reflective 'narratives of practice' of the sort being discussed here, which can be critically examined in terms of knowledge transmission. This shortage can be attributed to problems around the conceptualization of research for and from practice. The question of what constitutes acceptable research in the context of professional practice is therefore the focus of the next section.

HOW CAN THE KNOWLEDGE BASE OF A PROFESSION BE EXPANDED?

As we have seen in the preceding chapter, there are a number of conflicting groups with an interest in defining the knowledge base for professional practice. For individual learners, knowledge is personally constructed and owned, and tends to be transmitted in informal ways to fellow practitioners, when it can be articulated at all.

At the level of the professional body, there is a need for some formal definition of knowledge in order to make decisions about what level of knowledge is necessary for admission to membership of the profession. For the wider community, there is a requirement for still more formal knowledge to be disseminated in ways that can be examined by those outside the profession. Such an examination might be carried out by the NHS as evidence upon which decisions to fund particular types of healthcare will be taken, or by universities as part of the production and extension of research knowledge, which is seen as central to their role.

For the individual practitioner, one element of professionalism has to be the way that personal knowledge is related to more public forms of knowledge. This should be seen as a two-way process. Continuous professional development, as we have seen, is one of the markers of professional identity. Professionals constantly update themselves with developments in the field. So too the production of a distinctive knowledge base, another determinant of professional identity, has ultimately to be seen as the responsibility of the practitioners who make up the profession. This suggests some sort of dialectic process between the micro and the macro level of the profession, and between the profession and wider society, focused on the extension of knowledge. The passing back of personal knowledge into the practitioner community is part of the professional role of the individual. The report of the Herbal Medicine Regulatory Working Group (HMRWG 2003) made a series of recommendations around continuous professional development.

There is a relationship between continuous professional development and the dissemination of professional knowledge. The production of published research, the abstracting of theory from practice, is perhaps the most visible form of an activity that also includes the supervision and mentoring of more junior colleagues, the maintenance of one's own stance as a reflective practitioner and the transmission of knowledge through anecdote, story and narratives of practice (Benner 1984, Hunter 1986, 1989, Lave & Wenger 1991).

Conflicting conceptions of research in healthcare professions

It is possible to define three ways in which theory is generated from practice, and thus propositional knowledge is developed out of the personal and process knowledge of practitioners. For many professions, there is a tension between these different ways of knowing (Cribb & Bignold 1999).

The first of these methods is known as evidence-based practice (after Weinstein & Fineberg 1980). This utilizes both a research and policy perspective and a practitioner perspective. However, it incorporates a hierarchical model that privileges controlled trials and meta-analyses of controlled trials over other research methods and over generally accepted but untrialled practices in common use.

This approach to research has advocates and critics (Ernst 1994, Vickers 1997), with some pointing out that the majority of healthcare practices in use cannot be backed up by this sort of evidence base (the NHS research and development policy having been established as recently as 1991). Particular concern is voiced about such methods by holistic practitioners, who question the methodological premise that complex human issues of illness and well-being can be tested with methods that control out most of the variables. Alternative ways of conducting large-scale clinical trials are advocated by such commentators (Fitter and Thomas 1997, Thomas and Fitter 1997).

The second sort of theoretical understanding is that generated by people outside the profession, these being mostly usually located in a university. Here the emphasis may be in particular on the opportunity offered to generate new insights through cross-disciplinary understandings and inter- or multidisciplinary approaches. For example, much of the work in education on professional knowledge is being developed within psychological understandings of cognition. In the case of healthcare, there is an increased emphasis on the social and cultural nature of health, with a related movement to understanding and preventing illness before it occurs, rather than developing and refining treatments (Gaier 1998). This sort of research draws on sociological and psychological approaches to research.

The third, and most problematic, type of research activity is that focused on practice. Practice-based knowledge is advocated as a rich source of both personal and process knowledge (Benner 1984, Fish 1998, Moch 1990). However, the methods to be employed for capturing and disseminating such knowledge tend to be underconceptualized. Fish (1998) talks about constructing narratives to capture the 'artistry of practice', but is short of examples about how such research would be conducted.

Within the field of nursing there are a number of discussions and examples of this (Silva 1977, Swanson-Kauffman 1986). However, such accounts can be criticized on the basis of being 'merely' descriptive. While there is recognition that the examination of accounts of good practice by senior practitioners, or the skilled recognition of one or two cases that disprove a current theory, are part of the way that new knowledge is shared and developed, there are few large-scale attempts to employ such strategies as a specific contribution to formal knowledge.

An example of the reluctance to use this sort of experience in the formation of public knowledge is cited by Hunter (1986):

"Although the six cases he had seen were sufficient evidence, the Australian physician who established the teratogenic properties of thalidomide introduced the matter at a public meeting with an apology:

'As a scientist' he said 'I have no grounds for speaking. As a human being I cannot keep silent."

(Hunter 1986, p. 624)

Barnett (1994) argues that the more appropriate forms of knowledge for the future will be those that combine academic knowledge of the kind that constitutes an evidence base with more personal forms of knowing, and gives the greatest value to those that synthesize both approaches. He argues for an eclectic approach that does not favour one epistemology over another, but recognizes the limitations of all approaches. He calls this epistemology 'reflective knowing':

"Reflective knowing is relaxed about forms of knowing: it does not strike a fixed position about favoured epistemologies but accepts that all kinds of knowing can help us to understand our worlds better. At the same time, it adopts an ironic stance in relation to all forms of knowing. It knows that all forms of knowing are partial and so keeps a jaundiced eye on them all. No one form is allowed a privileged status. Science is not granted special favours; and nor is practical know-how."

(Barnett 1994, p. 180)

So, in healthcare, there are three loci for research into professional practice. These are the bodies that have an interest in safety and efficacy (i.e. health professionals), the universities, which have an interest in the extension and validation of knowledge, and the profession. The profession has an interest at both the level of the macro organization and, crucially, at the level of the practitioner with an interest in improving service to clients. Although it can be argued that it is this last grouping that has the greatest stake in formalizing the distinctive knowledge base that characterizes a given professional practice, this group tends to be more fragmented and less powerful than the first two groups.

Some of this can be attributed to issues around power and resources. However, it must also be recognized that the orientation to research and the generation of formal theory is something that needs to be embedded through the structures of professional education, as inherent in professional values. A research agenda shaped by professional values and concerns will look very different to one shaped by the interests of academics or healthcare professionals.

Eraut (1994) argues:

"A much broader framework is needed for studying the creation of professional knowledge; and the situation looks very different if we move the academic researcher from the centre of the universe . . . knowledge use and knowledge creation cannot be easily separated" (p. 54)

He goes on to argue that the problem with this kind of knowledge is that it may not be formulated clearly, and is unlikely to be disseminated widely. This leads to the problem of how practitioners can be encouraged to take a systematic approach to researching and learning from their own practice. We have seen above that Barnett (1994) advocates a synthesis of practical and academic knowledge, but the difficulty comes in finding mechanisms to assist practitioners in realizing their personal knowledge in some sort of public professional way.

Relationships between researchers and practitioners

There are a number of ways that universities can assist with this process. Some commentators feel there is a far greater role to be played by universities in continuous professional development, and in the extension of continuous professional development (an essentially private benefit) into research (a social benefit). Such commentators (Becher 1999, Solomon & Tresman 1999) would tend to construe professional development broadly, employing such methods as action research.

In a more formal way, universities can collaborate with practitioners in research activity, which serves the dual purpose of improving practice and developing more abstract theory. Huberman (1999) suggests that, although the ways in which the knowledge will be put to use differ, both researchers and practitioners benefit through sustained interactions between the academy and the practice context.

At its most productive, this way of constructing knowledge will feed back into the preparation of the next generation of practitioners. If there is a sustained dialogue between practitioners and researchers, which involves sharing ideas about the way knowledge is developed and, to some extent, collaborating in the construction of knowledge, both parties should end up with a more explicit understanding of the problems of knowledge and the interface between theory and practice. This will inform the teaching in both the university and the practicum setting. Brew (1999) argues:

"By drawing attention to underlying assumptions about the nature of knowledge and how these have been affecting both research and teaching, while ideas about teaching and research have changed and while ideas about knowledge have changed, it should now be clear that the relationships between teaching and research are dynamic and context driven."

(Brew 1999, p. 296)

However, less happily, these changing ideas about knowledge, learning and teaching, and the different perspectives of practitioner and teacher/researcher, can also prove to be a barrier to the next generation of practitioners. Issues of power and status may interfere to the detriment of the student experience and the construction of knowledge (Brew 1999, Burwood 1999). Insufficient attention may be paid to the ways students may themselves contribute to knowledge construction, particularly perhaps in adult learning groups with considerable prior life knowledge (Richardson 1994). Providers of such courses may be led by market models, rather than a demand-led vision of learning and knowledge production (Becher 1999).

What is important is the appropriation and transformation by learners of the discourse of their profession. This implies a two-way transformational relationship between the academic and the professional practitioner, part of the dialectic between the profession itself and the wider structures of society. This ideal may not be widely shared (Burwood 1999, Brew 1999, Solomon & Tresman 1999), and in Section Three of this volume we will consider some of the areas for conflict between professionals in higher education, other professional groupings and the individual practitioner who is the learner.

CONCLUSION

In this chapter, we have discussed the ways in which individual professionals learn their profession. We have seen that there are different sorts of knowledge for professional practice, and that the ability to access and use these different ways of knowing is itself a skill that a practitioner needs to acquire. The development and use of professional knowledge in practice is therefore a process that will take place across a professional's life. Professional knowledge is ultimately built upon the values and beliefs that underpin practice, and are often acquired as a professional is socialized into the mores of the profession. This sort of learning can be fostered by the adoption of a reflective orientation, which allows for a personal exploration and construction of knowledge.

For the profession of herbal medicine, at the historical moment at which it enters into a formal and acknowledged relationship with society through statutory self-regulation, education and knowledge creation thus become critical areas for examination. On the one hand, there exists the pressure to adapt to normative theories of education, the development of the evidence base and the nature of professional knowledge. On the other, for individual practitioners a clear sense of what is 'different' and 'other' about learning, education and research in herbal medicine is a key component in maintaining professional identity at a time of major change. Thus, as we shall see, the recommendations of the HMRWG were particularly problematic when debated or discussed by individuals or small groups of practitioners in relation to their own practice.

References

Argyris C, Schon D A 1974 Theory in practice: increasing professional effectiveness. Jossey Bass, San Francisco

Barnett R 1994 The limits of competence: knowledge, higher education and society. Society for Research into Higher Education/Open University Press, Buckingham

Becher T 1999 Universities and mid-career professionals: the policy potential. Higher Education Quarterly 53(2):156–172

Benner P 1984 From novice to expert: excellence and power in clinical nursing practice. Addison-Wesley, New York

Brew A 1999 Research and teaching: changing relationships in a changing context. Studies in Higher Education 24(3):291–301

Burwood S 1999 Liberation philosophy. Teaching in Higher Education 4(4):447–460

Carper B 1978 Fundamental ways of knowing in nursing. Advances in Nursing Science 1(1):13–23

Cribb A, Bignold, S 1999 Towards a reflexive medical school: the hidden curriculum and medical education research. Studies in Higher Education 24(2):195–209

Dreyfus H L, Dreyfus S E 1986 Mind over machine: the power of human intuition and expertise in the era of the computer. Blackwell, Oxford

Eraut M 1994 Developing professional knowledge and competence. Falmer, London

Eraut M 1995 Schon shock: a case for reframing reflection-in-action? Teachers and Teaching: Theory and Practice 1(1):9–22

Eraut M 2000 Non-formal learning and tacit knowledge in professional work. British Journal of Educational Psychology 70:113–136

Eraut M, Alderton J, Boylan A et al 1995 Learning to use scientific knowledge in education and practicum settings: an evaluation of the contribution of the biological, behavioural and social sciences to pre-registration nursing and midwifery courses. English National Board for Nursing, Midwifery and Health Visiting, London

Eraut M, Alderton J, Cole G et al 1998 Development of knowledge and skills in employment. University of Sussex Institute of Education, Falmer, Sussex

Ernst E 1994 Acupuncture research: Where are the problems? Acupuncture in Medicine 12:93–97

Fish D 1998 Appreciating practice in the caring professions. Butterworth Heinemann, Oxford

Fitter M, Thomas K J 1997 Evaluating complementary therapies for use in the National Health Service: 'horses for courses', part 1: the design challenge. Complementary Therapies in Medicine 5:90–93

Gaier H 1998 A critique of the limiting consequences of current thinking in healthcare and proposals for the next millennium: reflections on the catallactics for integrated healthcare delivery. Journal of Alternative and Complementary Medicine 4(2):249–254

Gear J, McIntosh A, Squires G 1994 Informal learning in the professions. Department of Adult Education, University of Hull

Herbal Medicine Regulatory Working Group 2003 Recommendations on the regulation of herbal practitioners. Prince of Wales's Foundation for Integrated Health, London

Huberman M 1999 The mind is its own place: the influence of sustained interactivity with practitioners on educational researchers. Harvard Educational Review 69(3):289–319

Hunter K M 1986 'There was this one guy. . .'; the uses of anecdote in medicine. Perspectives in Biology and Medicine 29(4):619–630

Hunter K M 1989 A science of individuals; medicine and casuistry. Journal of Medicine and Philosophy 14:193–212

Johns C 1995 Framing learning through reflection within Carper's fundamental ways of knowledge in nursing. Journal of Advanced Nursing 22:226–234

Kolb D A 1984 Experiential learning: experience as the source of learning and development. Prentice Hall, Englewood Cliffs

Lave J, Wenger E 1991 Situated learning: legitimate peripheral participation. Cambridge University Press, Cambridge

McIntyre D 1994 Preface. In: Eraut M (ed) Developing professional knowledge and competence. Falmer, London

Moch S 1990 Personal knowing: evolving research and practice. Scholarly Inquiry for Nursing Practice 4(2):155–165

Richardson J T E 1994 Mature students in higher education: 1. A literature survey on approaches to studying. Studies in Higher Education 19(3):309–325

Ryle G 1949 The concept of mind. Hutchinson, London

Schon D A 1987 Educating the reflective practitioner. Jossey-Bass, San Francisco

Silva M C 1977 Philosophy, science, theory: interrelationships and implications for nursing research. Image 9(3):59–63

Solomon J, Tresman S 1999 A model for continued professional development: knowledge, belief and action. Journal of In-Service Education 25(2):307–319

Swanson-Kauffman K M 1986 A combined qualitative methodology for nursing research. Advances In Nursing Science 8:58–69

Thomas K J, Fitter M J 1997 Evaluating complementary therapies for use in the National Health Service: 'horses for courses', part 2: alternative research strategies. Complementary Therapies in Medicine 5:94–98

Vickers A 1997 How should we research unconventional therapies? International Journal of the Assessment of Health Care 13:111–121

Weinstein M C, Fineberg H V 1980 Clinical decision analysis. WB Saunders, Philadelphia

The traditions of herbal medicine

Chinese herbal medicine:
the history and context to statutory self-regulation

3

Nick Lampert

OVERVIEW

Chinese herbal medicine is one modality within the broad tradition of Chinese medicine, which also includes acupuncture, massage (*tuina*), breathing exercises (*qi gong*) and dietary therapy. This tradition has evolved over two or three millennia and today is still practised throughout much of South-East Asia. It is state sponsored in hospitals throughout China, where it enjoys a pragmatic working relationship with orthodox Western medicine. In the UK, Chinese herbal medicine is a relative newcomer, having developed rather later than acupuncture. However, it has grown greatly in popularity since the late 1980s, with an increase in the number of Western practitioners trained in the tradition, and a rapid expansion in the number of Chinese medicine outlets staffed primarily by practitioners from China. In the great majority of cases these practitioners, whether trained in the West or in China, are also qualified in acupuncture and work with the two modalities in an integrated way.

By way of introduction to Chinese herbal medicine and its current position in the UK, this chapter will examine briefly:

- the historical background
- key underlying concepts
- approaches to diagnosis
- forms of treatment
- questions of efficacy and safety
- current forms of regulation of Chinese herbal medicine in the UK .

EARLY HISTORY

Within its very long history, many different approaches to diagnosis and treatment have evolved within Chinese medicine. Hence, as has been persuasively argued in a recent work (Scheid 2002), it is more accurate to speak of Chinese medicines in the plural than of a single entity. This variety of forms can be seen in the presence of folk medicine alongside elite medicine, in the emergence of distinct styles of practice within medical families, and in a constant evolution of the tradition in response to new medical challenges in different parts of China. At the same time, there developed from very early times a strong literary tradition, which provided the basis for a definite continuity, and has allowed a set of core concepts about health and disease to be shared by practitioners of Chinese medicine around the world.

The literary tradition within Chinese medicine provides a written record going back to the third century BCE. Famous texts from the Chinese tradition include the *Yellow Emperor's inner classic* (*Huang Di Nei Jing*) compiled between 200 BCE and 100 CE and the *Divine husbandsman's classic of the materia medica* (*Shen Nong Ben Cao Jing*) from the later Han dynasty (25–220 CE). The *Discussion of cold-induced disorders* (*Shang han Lun*), written about 220 CE by one of China's most renowned herbal doctors, Zhang Zhong Jing, outlines the treatment of various conditions arising from exterior causes. Several of its formulas are still in use today. Sun Si Miao (581–682 CE), another famous physician and scholar who was versed in both Buddhist and Daoist philosophies, devised in his *Thousand ducat formulas (Qian Jin Yao Fang)* and his supplement to the *Thousand ducat formulas (Qian Jin Yi Fang)* an extensive repertory of prescriptions that similarly influence Chinese herbal practice to the present day. The *Materia medica arranged according to drug descriptions and technical aspects (Ben Cao Gang Mu)* by Li Shi Zhen published in 1596 was the outcome of 40 years of work. This book contains 52 chapters describing 1893 medicinal substances. Among other things, Li Shi Zhen demonstrated the connection between sweets and tooth decay and described occupational illnesses such as lead poisoning. In the late Ming and Qing dynasties, new theories concerning the treatment of disease were developed by five famous doctors: Wu You Ke, Ye Tian Shi, Xue Sheng Bai, Wu Ju Tong and Wang Meng Ying. All these physicians were adherents of the 'Warm diseases theory' (*Wen Bing Xue*), which addressed the treatment of rapidly transmitted infectious disease. These are just a few highlights from an immensely rich medical legacy (Bensky & Barolet 1990, Bensky & Gamble1993).

MODERN TIMES

In modern times, Chinese herbal medicine has continued to develop as part of what is now called Traditional Chinese Medicine (TCM), and it has taken its place within the Chinese healthcare system alongside Western medicine. After taking power in 1949, the Communist Party encouraged the use of Chinese herbs as a cost-effective alternative to expensive Western drugs and continued to publish materia medica. For example, in 1977 the *Encyclopaedia of traditional Chinese medicinal substances* (*Zhong Yao Da Zi Dian*) representing 25 years of research was published by the Jiangsu College of New Medicine. This monumental work contained 5767 entries, a compilation of China's herbal tradition to that time.

Before the Communist era, Chinese medicine was practised in private clinics and hospitals and transmitted through apprenticeships or private schools. From the 1950s it began to be systematized and taught in state-controlled institutions, and now appears in translation as 'Traditional Chinese Medicine'. This process of systematization was influenced by two opposing factors: on the one hand the drive to modernize and to follow Western models, on the other the desire to accommodate the professional agenda of Chinese medicine and to protect the image of a distinct cultural heritage (Scheid 2002).

The tensions between the claims of the traditional medicine and the forces of westernization were already present in the Republican period, but appeared again after the Communist revolution. At first, state support for Chinese medicine was only lukewarm and the goal was to assimilate it to Western medicine. This was in effect a continuation of Guomindang policies, which had been hostile to the TCM Chinese medical tradition. Later, in the mid 1950s, there was a shift in policy, driven by the desire to use all available resources, to avoid excessive dependence on imported technology and drugs and to limit the ideological influence of Western medicine practitioners. As a result a number of key practitioners who had stood up for Chinese medicine in the 1920s and 1930s were able to exercise a strong influence on its development under state socialism. The Academy of Chinese Medicine was established, Chinese medicine was integrated into the larger hospitals and the national insurance scheme and separate Chinese medicine hospitals and training colleges were set up.

This process was conducted under the direct supervision of the Ministry of Health and was accompanied by the search for new teaching methods that would impose greater coherence on the tradition. That led to serious concerns among some practitioners that the vitality of the tradition was being undermined. However, those disputes were brought to a halt in 1965, with a programme of mass action and attacks on Western-style professionalism. During the ensuing Cultural Revolution period, formal Chinese medicine education ceased, the Academy of Chinese Medicine was closed, and the publication of medical journals was suspended. The Chinese medicine sector lost 30% of its manpower between 1959 and 1977 (while Western medicine manpower increased four times). Renowned practitioners were branded 'forces of evil', subject to abuse and sometimes physical attack and many were banished to out-of-the-way provinces. Private practices and pharmacies were destroyed; classical medical texts were burned.

In the late 1970s, with the fall of the 'Gang of Four', the pursuit of 'socialism with Chinese characteristics' allowed Chinese medicine to re-establish its position in hospital-based services, with renewed official support for specialist knowledge. The Ministry of Health affirmed the independence of the Chinese medicine sector while at the same time strongly encouraging modernization. In the 1980s it was agreed that Western medicine, Chinese medicine and integrated Chinese/Western medicine (in reality a subfield of Chinese medicine) would constitute the three pillars of healthcare.

Within this scheme of things, Chinese medicine has been a relatively small player. However, it is still deeply embedded in the healthcare system, with a network of TCM training institutions, and the provision of TCM hospitals and TCM departments within Western medicine hospitals. Westernization has affected the manner in which Chinese medicine is researched, taught and delivered, but the tradition remains very much part of the medical landscape. In certain ways it has even been strengthened by more recent social and economic reforms, because of the major effort to expand the international market for TCM products (Scheid 2002).

In addition to its continuing strength in China itself, Chinese medicine has been strikingly successful in establishing a position as a complementary and alternative therapy in the West, especially in the UK and the USA. The herbal side of Chinese medicine came relatively late to the UK in comparison with acupuncture. At a time – the late 1980s – when acupuncture was already quite well established, Chinese herbal medicine was only beginning to make its presence felt. This was a very different situation from that in China itself, where herbal medicine has occupied a far larger place than acupuncture within the domain of TCM as a whole. However, there was a significant expansion in the provision of Chinese herbal medicine in the UK from the late 1980s. This was partly due to an increase in graduates emerging from UK colleges of Chinese medicine, but to a greater extent was the result of a growth in the number of Chinese medicine outlets in the 'high street' sector, generally staffed by practitioners who had been recruited from China and came to work in the UK and sometimes to settle.

PRINCIPLES OF TCM

Underlying TCM are the three fundamental concepts of Yin, Yang and Qi. Box 3.1 details these ideas.

Box 3.1   Key concepts: Yin–Yang and Qi

Despite the great variety of styles of practice that may be encountered within the field of Chinese medicine, there are a number of concepts relating to health and disease that are likely to inform the practice of the great majority of Chinese medicine practitioners around the world. In the broadest terms, good health is seen as a state in which a person has optimum vitality and in which the various functions needed to maintain that vitality are unimpeded. Ill health is due to a loss of that vitality or to some form of impediment to those functions, or both. Good health furthermore requires a balance, which is represented by the core idea of *Yin–Yang*, a concept drawn from a school of thought that came to be central to the Chinese medical tradition.

The polarity of Yin–Yang represents the mutual dependence of all things. In the context of human life, health and disease, this can be understood in the following way. Any form of life depends on substance and activity. Substance is Yin; it is the stuff our bodies are made of: bones, muscles, internal organs, blood, fluid and so on. Activity is Yang; it is movement or transformation, including the transformation required to repair and build body tissue. The relationship between them can be likened to the wax and flame of a candle.

The wax is the Yin aspect (substance), the flame is the Yang (activity, transformation, heat). They are mutually dependent. You need wax as fuel for the activity (hence wax is consumed by the flame), while you need a process of transformation in order to create wax. The comparison is not complete, because a candle has a fixed amount of substance. Once the wax is consumed the candle ceases to burn, while human beings continue to take in nourishment in order to keep the flame alive. Still, our life is also limited, the substance is consumed with age and the flame eventually goes out.

In the most general terms, the way to preserve health and achieve longevity is to maintain a harmony of Yin and Yang. This means creating a balance between substance and activity that will maximize 'Qi' (pronounced 'Chee', hard to translate but close to energy or vitality), which is necessary for all life functions, and will ensure that Qi flows freely, without stasis. On one side is nourishment, rest and calm (Yin); on the other is activity/movement/ transformation (Yang). If the Yin is in excess relative to the Yang (let us say through a life of overeating and underexercising), there is a slowing down, a stasis: the flame is reduced. If there is an excess of Yang relative to Yin (for example through a chronically overactive lifestyle, with inadequate rest and recovery), the substance is too quickly depleted: the flame burns too fast. Either way the Qi/vitality/energy will be compromised (diminished or blocked), leading to dysfunction and disease.

In Chinese thought, achieving harmony of Yin and Yang is not only, and not even primarily, a matter for medicine. Medical intervention can help to redress imbalances, to relieve suffering and to fend off disease. Yet the ways in which life is lived are more important, including appropriate diet and exercise, work and rest, emotional states and attitudes of mind. These basic elements of traditional wisdom, discovered anew by modern health education, help to keep the role of the physician in proper perspective.

Diagnosing patterns of disharmony

The Yin–Yang polarity deeply informs the Chinese medicine tradition, and establishes a way of thinking in which component elements, though they can be distinguished, are inseparable parts of a whole. Whereas modern biomedicine is typically concerned with disease categories that can be isolated and identified from laboratory tests, Chinese medicine describes patterns of disharmony. The interest is not only in the symptoms and signs associated with a specific area of dysfunction, but in the relationship of these symptoms to the wider pattern of which they are a part, and which give them diagnostic meaning. In this sense Chinese medicine is concerned with the whole person (Kaptchuk 1983).

The description of patterns of disharmony does not stand in opposition to conventional diagnosis or objective tests, the importance of which is well understood. In practice, the great majority of patients seen by Chinese medicine practitioners in the UK have been diagnosed conventionally, and any competent practitioner will know when it is inappropriate to go ahead without a prior conventional diagnosis. Furthermore, practitioners will distinguish between alternative and complementary treatment. Chinese medicine may be used as an alternative where a condition has been conventionally diagnosed but the treatment is not helping and has been abandoned, or where there is no convincing conventional diagnosis or treatment. It is also frequently used in a complementary way alongside orthodox approaches, typically where patients are seeking ways to reduce dependence on conventional drugs.

Diagnosis is the identification of a pattern of disharmony displayed by the individual patient, based on four main methods: observing, listening, questioning and palpating. A disharmony may be read in a number of ways. From one perspective, it may involve a deficiency or dysfunction in one or more of the 'Organs', in particular the Spleen, Liver, Heart, Lungs or Kidneys. These 'Organs' are not to be confused with the anatomical organs of biomedicine: they refer rather to spheres of function. For example in Chinese medicine the 'Spleen' is concerned with the 'transformation and transportation' of food and drink. It has been likened to the pancreas, but such comparisons obscure more than they reveal. The key thing is the function, which is the digestion and assimilation of food. A strong Spleen means a strong digestion, which is the basis for good energy, good appetite, normal bowel pattern and freedom from digestive discomfort. If there is a deficiency of the Spleen, this might manifest as tiredness (the energy from food is not being efficiently extracted and transported around the body), loss of appetite (absorption has slowed down), loose stools (food is inadequately digested) or abdominal discomfort or pain (poor functioning leads to stasis).

Most of the 'Organs' do include the organ suggested by the English term, and the Chinese Lungs, Kidneys, and Heart are indeed associated with respiratory, urinary and circulatory functions. However, it is best not to assume anything about the relationship between the Chinese Organ and the anatomical entity. Hence to say that there is a 'Liver disharmony' or a 'Kidney deficiency' does not mean that there is anything wrong with the liver or kidneys in the conventional sense (though there may be).

Another perspective in diagnosis involves identifying patterns according to the presence of pathogenic factors. Such factors, which are not to be thought of as microbes, are described in terms derived from the natural world, namely Heat, Cold, Dampness, Wind, Dryness, together with varieties of Toxin and disease-causing products of the body described as Blood stasis and Phlegm. These patterns may have an external origin in climate or environment – for example, a damp house or damp working conditions may lead to a Damp condition affecting the joints; a hot environment may aggravate a Hot condition affecting the skin. However, Dampness or Heat do not refer to causative agents as such; rather it is the pattern as a whole that is defined as Damp or Hot.

Other forms of diagnosis are also used, for example differentiating the 'level' at which the disease is found, which may be outer or inner, with other distinctions at the inner level. There are agreed criteria for identifying disharmonies at the different levels, and this may in important ways affect the treatment strategy.

Alongside the identification of patterns of disharmony, much attention is also given to aetiology (the origins of disease). The origins of disease are broadly categorized as listed in Box 3.2.

Box 3.2   The origins of disease

- *External:* these are again described as Heat, Cold, Dampness, Dryness, Wind, but in this case referring to outside forces impinging on the person
- *Internal, relating mainly to the emotional sphere:* seven emotions (joy, anger, worry, pensiveness, sadness, fear and fright) appear in the Chinese medical tradition, and each can take a pathological form, thus becoming a source of disharmony
- *Neither external nor internal:* these factors include diet, imbalances of work and rest, and sexual factors
- *Other origins:* including trauma, burns, bites and parasites. Inherited and congenital factors, although not typically included in textbook accounts, are also recognized

---

TREATING WITH CHINESE HERBAL MEDICINE

The art of treatment with Chinese herbal medicine is to choose a formula, a combination of herbs, that matches the pattern of disharmony of the individual, and to modify the formula in order to accommodate changes in the course of treatment and, if necessary, revisions in diagnosis. If the condition is diagnosed as a malfunction of one or more of the Organs, then this is addressed by 'supplementing' that function or eliminating blockages that impede it. If the disharmony is due to the predominance of a certain pathogenic factor, the treatment will require eliminating or resolving it in some way so as to restore balance or strengthen some aspect of the person's vitality in order to assist in that process, or both.

The Chinese materia medica contains several hundred commonly used ingredients, including roots, stems, flowers, leaves and barks, together with some non-plant ingredients. The choice of an appropriate formula is the choice of a combination of herbs or other medicinals with certain properties. Properties refer, first, to 'taste' or 'flavour': sweet, sour, bitter, pungent, salty or bland. Secondly, they describe temperature: hot, warm, cool, cold, neutral. This is not a thermometer reading, but a quality that has been identified from its observed physiological effect. Hence ginger is warming, mint is cooling. Thirdly, substances may be described as having an outward or inward movement; for example some pungent substances help to 'sweat out' a disease, whereas sour substances have an inward action by virtue of their astringent properties. In a further dimension, medicinals are seen as affecting particular channels or meridians, although this aspect is more important for acupuncture than for herbal medicine.

The materia medica is then grouped into broad categories in accordance with physiological action. For example there are medicinals that:

- 'release the exterior', i.e. treat the early stages of disease caused by external agents
- 'clear Heat' through their cooling and usually bitter properties
- treat Damp-Heat by clearing Heat and drying Dampness
- 'warm the interior'
- 'drain Dampness' through their diuretic action
- 'transform Dampness' by virtue of their warm and aromatic properties
- 'transform Phlegm'
- 'regulate Qi' by treating certain Qi stagnation
- 'invigorate Blood' by treating Blood stagnation
- 'calm the spirit'
- 'supplement' one or another form of deficiency.

Chinese medicinals are rarely prescribed as 'simples' or single remedies. They are combined into formulas that will typically contain 10 or more ingredients. The principle is that a balance of ingredients with certain properties is matched to a pattern of disharmony, allowing for great flexibility in addressing the individual characteristics of the patient and changes that occur during the course of treatment.

The history of Chinese herbal medicine is marked by the development of numerous formulas, now designated 'classical', developed over the centuries by a number of brilliant practitioners whose work has become part of a rich heritage. These formulas were often designed to treat disease patterns that belonged to particular historical periods, and very many are not now used in their original form. However, some remain directly relevant to the practice of herbal medicine today, while others may be used for purposes other than those for which they were originally intended. Others again are used for teaching purposes because they illustrate especially well the general principles that govern the building of formulas.

Chinese herbal medicine may be prescribed in a number of ways. The main traditional method is the tea. A combination of loose herbs is prepared for the patient, who makes a tea or decoction, a water extract produced by simmering, and drinks it twice a day. The most commonly used items in the materia medica can now also be obtained in the form of concentrated powders. These are often preferred to teas for reasons of convenience and better compliance. However, teas retain definite advantages, because the ingredients are cooked together, creating a potential for synergy between the ingredients (as happens in the cooking of a soup or stew). The raw ingredients can also be prepared in a number of ways before making the tea, for example by dry-frying or charring, or frying with honey, vinegar or salt. This changes the property of the raw material, strengthening or moderating a particular action.

In addition, a wide range of formulas is available in tablet form. These are very convenient and frequently used, but lack the flexibility of individually prepared prescriptions. External *preparations* are also made, including creams, ointments and washes for skin conditions, and compresses for traumatized tissue.

Conditions suitable for treatment with Chinese herbal medicine

The possible uses of Chinese herbal medicine are very wide, but a number of conditions may be singled out, as listed in Box 3.3.

Box 3.3   Conditions suitable for treatment with Chinese herbal medicine

- Dermatological, including eczema and psoriasis
- Respiratory, including asthma, bronchitis, rhinitis and sinusitis
- Gastrointestinal, in particular irritable bowel syndrome and other functional gastrointestinal disorders
- Gynaecological, including premenstrual syndrome, painful periods, menopausal syndrome, endometriosis, and some forms of infertility
- Urinary, including chronic cystitis
- Rheumatological, including rheumatoid and osteoarthritis
- Headaches
- Chronic fatigue syndromes
- Anxiety and depression
- Hepatitis and HIV (some promising results have been obtained for treatment of Hepatitis C, and supportive treatment may be beneficial in the case of HIV)
- Metabolic, including supportive treatment for diabetes and thyroid conditions

---

EFFICACY AND EVIDENCE

A very large body of research exists on Chinese herbal medicine, including clinical trials covering a wide range of conditions, and extensive pharmacological studies. The bulk of it has been undertaken in China and elsewhere in the Far East. A large portion of the Chinese studies takes the form of clinical outcome studies, though controlled trials (in particular comparing Chinese medicine with pharmaceutical drugs) have increasingly become the norm (Dharmananda 1997). A review of Chinese controlled studies from the 1980s and 1990s revealed a number of problems, including possible biases deriving from study design, from publication policy and the general absence of any discussion of randomization and blinding (Department of Human Services 1996). Hence the position is that, although Chinese herbal medicine is deeply grounded in traditional use and has demonstrated great strength around the world, much remains to be done in meeting internationally agreed research standards.

Those randomized, placebo-controlled trials using Chinese herbal medicine that have so far been conducted have shown promising results. These include trials on the treatment of non-exudative atopic eczema (Sheehan & Atherton 1992, Sheehan et al 1992), hepatitis C (Batey et al 1998) and irritable bowel syndrome (Bensoussan et al 1998). In terms of clinical trial methodology, the challenge for research is to combine rigorous design with the flexibility required in treating the individual patient, which is a necessary condition if the practice of Chinese herbal medicine is to be fully tested. In these and other ways to be discussed elsewhere in this book (see Chapter 10), Chinese and other traditional forms of medicine offer a challenge for research design and generate wider questions about what constitutes valid knowledge.

SAFETY

The available figures suggest that the incidence of adverse events from herbal medicines in general is low (Shaw et al 1997[1]), and herbal medicines appear very safe by comparison with pharmaceutical drugs. However, all medicines, whether pharmaceutical or herbal, must be treated with respect. As emphasized elsewhere in this publication, 'natural' does not mean safe. Medicines that have the power to do good also have the potential to cause harm if improperly used, and appropriate use must be learned through rigorous professional training. These issues were highlighted in the Chinese medicine tradition from very early times. Clear rules were laid down about dosage (bearing in mind that toxicity is to a large extent a matter of dosage), about ingredients that might safely be used long term, those that should be used short term or with special care, and those that were to be avoided in pregnancy. The special preparation of some ingredients was also developed from very early on, so as to soften the harsh effects of certain ingredients. Furthermore, Chinese medicinal formulas are built on the idea of balance, in which the one-sided effects of some ingredients are modified by the addition of others with contrasting qualities.

These are important safeguards, which require thorough learning. In addition, some further safety issues have arisen in recent years that have tended to put the spotlight on herbal medicine in general and Chinese medicine in particular. These issues are listed in Box 3.4.

The first three points in Box 3.4 highlight the importance of adequate professional skills and knowledge of the law, with regular updating of practitioners through their professional bodies, and CPD. The last two points concern issues of quality assurance, since practitioners rely on their suppliers for access to authentic and unadulterated products. They are being addressed through the development of 'good manufacturing practice', through ensuring independent audit of suppliers, and linking practitioners to such suppliers through regulation of the profession. (For discussion of product regulation see Chapter 9.)

Box 3.4   Safety issues

- *The predictable toxicity of certain ingredients:* the most notable example involving Chinese herbal medicine has arisen from the use of plant species of the genus *Aristolochia*. Aristolochic acids have been shown to be potentially very toxic for the kidneys (EMEA 2001). Aristolochias have therefore been banned for use in unlicensed medicines in the UK, together with the use of certain non-aristolochic species that may be confused with them (Medicines (Aristolochia and Mu Tong etc.) (Prohibition) Order 2001)
- *'Idiosyncratic' reactions* (so called because they are unpredictable), in particular affecting the liver. Such reactions can occur with any form of medicine, and are rare both with pharmaceutical drugs and herbs. The key thing is careful monitoring of the patient in case any suspect symptoms occur; a fundamental part of competent practice. As soon as such symptoms appear, treatment will be stopped, liver tests can be carried out, and lasting damage can be prevented
- *Possible adverse herb–drug interactions:* the widespread use of Chinese medicine in parallel with conventional medication, without apparent ill effects, suggests that the potential for problems from such interactions is quite limited. However, some examples are now well documented (Medicines Control Agency 2002), and it is essential to be cautious. Both herbal practitioners and medics need to be aware of all treatments that a patient is using and to take this into account where appropriate. This has extended the range of safety concerns and now forms part of Chinese medicine training
- *The sale of remedies:* an example being that of skin creams that purport to be herbal but contain prescription-only drugs (e.g. steroids), or contain other illegal substances (e.g. heavy metals)
- *Failure by suppliers to ensure the correct identification* of herbs or herbal products

---

REGULATION OF CHINESE HERBAL MEDICINE IN THE UK

As indicated earlier, Chinese herbal medicine developed in the UK somewhat later than acupuncture, but began to grow in importance in the 1980s. The first association with a specific remit to regulate Chinese herbal medicine, the Register of Chinese Herbal Medicine (RCHM), was set up in 1987. This was followed by the establishment of the Association of Traditional Chinese Medicine (ATCM) in 1994. A third organization, the British Society for Chinese Medicine, emerged briefly in 2001–2003, but then merged to become part of the ATCM at the end of 2003. These organizations have taken on the key role of protecting the public by upholding standards of training and ethical practice. They were represented on the Herbal Medicine Regulatory Working Group and have given consistent strong support to the statutory regulation of Chinese herbal medicine. At the time of writing they together represent about

1000 practitioners. However, it is estimated that at least as many practitioners as this (precise figures are not known), primarily within the 'high street' Chinese medicine outlets, remain unregulated.

Like other voluntary professional bodies, the RCHM and ATCM have carried out the dual function of upholding standards, while also defending and promoting the cause of Chinese medicine in the public domain. This is a sometimes difficult balancing act that is better tackled under a statutory system, where protection of the public belongs to the statutory body while promotional functions can be carried out by professional associations.

The range of work that has been conducted under voluntary regulation (here I am drawing on the work of the Register of Chinese Herbal Medicine) includes:

- establishing a list of affiliated training institutions whose graduates are entitled to automatic membership of the association
- developing a scheme for CPD, with a mentoring arrangement in the first 2 years of practice
- implementing a code of ethics and complaints procedures, together with a dispensary code for practitioners who run their own pharmacies
- communicating with members of the public seeking suitably qualified practitioners in their area, with other professional bodies and with the media
- publication of journals, with updates on professional, political and legal developments affecting Chinese herbal medicine, together with discussion pages, clinical studies and reviews
- preparation of quarterly abstracts on recent research (including research in the orthodox literature) dealing with safety and efficacy
- support for research projects on Chinese herbal medicine
- adoption of a 'yellow card' system to monitor adverse events
- establishing an approved suppliers scheme, which enables the association to recommend suppliers who have been through an independent audit of quality assurance, thus giving patients better protection against poor quality or illegal products
- support for the Chinese Herb Garden in Bristol, set up under the joint auspices of the University of Bristol and the Register of Chinese Herbal Medicine. This is doing important conservation work on which the future of Chinese herbal medicine will ultimately depend, and provides an educational resource for undergraduate and postgraduate courses on the materia medica
- close collaboration with the Chinese Medicinal Plant Authentication Centre at the Royal Botanic Gardens, Kew, which is engaged in pioneering work on the authentication of Chinese medicinal plants (Leon 2002)

- membership of the European Herbal Practitioners Association (EHPA) and full participation in the intensive work towards statutory self-regulation that was undertaken in the late 1990s and early 2000s under the auspices of the EHPA.

CONCLUSION

The activities described above testify to the presence of strong voluntary regulation for Chinese herbal medicine in the UK. However, this exists for only part of the sector, since significant numbers of practitioners remain outside these voluntary arrangements. Statutory regulation is, without doubt, the way forward, and both the RCHM and the ATCM have strongly supported this development, so long as the specific identity and culture of the profession are respected within that process. (For an extended discussion of this issue, see Chapter 10.)

Chinese herbal medicine is an enormously rich tradition that has much to offer in the treatment of many conditions, some of which have proved resistant to other forms of medicine. As this chapter has sought to describe, it works with particular diagnostic concepts and treatment methods, and these require mastery in their own terms. This highlights the importance of self-regulation within a statutory framework. The associations representing Chinese herbal medicine are committed to protecting patients through publicly recognized standards of competence and ethical practice, to the development of a stronger research base, and to a closer relationship with the NHS. At the same time they seek to establish a framework of regulation in which the distinctive language of description, diagnosis and treatment can find a legitimate place. It is in this way that Chinese herbal medicine will be able to realize its full potential contribution to contemporary healthcare in the UK.

References

Batey R G, Bensoussan A, Fan Y Y et al 1998 Preliminary report of a randomised, double blind placebo-controlled trial of a Chinese herbal medicine preparation CH-100 in the treatment of chronic hepatitis C. Journal of Gastroenterology and Hepatology 13:244–247

Bensky D, Barolet R 1990 Formulas and strategies. Eastland Press, Seattle

Bensky D, Gamble A 1993 Materia medica. Eastland Press, Seattle

Bensoussan A , Talley N J, Hing M et al 1998 Treatment of irritable bowel syndrome with Chinese herbal medicine. Journal of the American Medical Association 280:1585–1589

Department of Human Services 1996 Towards a safer choice: the practice of Chinese medicine in Australia. Public Health Division, Department of Human Services, Melbourne, Victoria

Dharmananda S 1997 Controlled clinical trials of Chinese herbal medicine: a review. Institute for Traditional Medicine, Oregon

EMEA Herbal Medicinal Products Working Party 2001 Position paper on risks associated with use of herbal products containing Aristolochia species. Online. Available: http://www.eudra.org/emea.html October 2004

Kaptchuk T 1983 Chinese medicine: the web that has no weaver. Rider, London

Leon C 2002 Chinese Medicinal Plants Authentication Centre. RCHM News, May
Medicines (Aristolochia and Mu Tong etc.) (Prohibition) Order 2001 Statutory
     Instrument 1841. Online. Available: http://www.mhra.gov.uk
Medicines Control Agency 2002 The safety of herbal medicinal products. HMSO,
     London
Nanjing College of Traditional Chinese Medicine, Shang Han Lun Research Group 1980
     Discussion on cold-induced diseases (*Shang Han Lun*) by Zhang Zhong Jing.
     Shanghai Scientific Publishing House, Shanghai, first published c. 220 CE.
Scheid V 2002 Chinese medicine in contemporary China: plurality and synthesis. Duke
     University Press, Durham NC
Sheehan M P, Atherton D J 1992 A controlled trial of traditional Chinese medicinal
     plants in widespread non-exudative atopic eczema. British Journal of
     Dermatology 126:179–184
Sheehan M P, Rustin M H, Atherton D J et al 1992 Efficacy of traditional Chinese
     herbal therapy in adult atopic dermatitis. Lancet 340:13–17
Shaw D, Leon C, Kolev S et al 1997 Traditional Remedies and Food Supplements. A
     five-year toxicological study (1991–1995). Drug Safety 17:342–356
1979 The Yellow Emperor's classic of internal medicine (*Huang Ti Nei Jing*). People's
     Health Publishing House, Beijing, first published c. 100 BCE.

NOTES

1. This study, undertaken by the National Poisons Unit (NPU), examined adverse
   events involving traditional medicines and food supplements. The NPU received
   1297 enquiries; however a link was identified as probable between exposure and
   reported adverse effects in just 38 of these cases. At the time, the Ministry of
   Agriculture, Fisheries and Food issued a press release (326/96), which stated that
   'The findings overall are reassuring as they do not indicate any significant health
   problems associated with most types of traditional remedies and dietary
   supplements.'

4

A brief history of traditional Tibetan medicine and its introduction to the United Kingdom

Katia Holmes and Ken Holmes (with Brion Sweeney)

OVERVIEW

This chapter looks at the development of traditional Tibetan medicine (TTM), emphasizing in particular the influence of Ayurvedic and Chinese medicine on its historical beginnings. This, it is argued, shows a 'translating' of cultural concepts that goes far beyond the mere technicalities of a system of medicine. Rather, the transmission of the practice of medicine between some of the great cultures of the world, in a process that stretched over many centuries, should be seen as a deep extension of human knowledge.

Within Tibet, as in India and China, there has always been a scholarly tradition of medicine. This meant that practices were recorded in written texts, and debated and developed in an iterative process between practitioners and scholars of different traditions, in different regions and countries.

This iterative process can be seen to have extended into modern times. This chapter records the ways in which TTM has come into the UK, and some of the tensions that this has caused within the practitioner community. Such tensions arise from differences in training practice between the three great universities of Tibetan medicine in Asia, and between ideas of education there and in the UK system of higher education. In describing the ways such differences were reconciled, the chapter ends with a vision of an integrated model of progression between modern and traditional programmes of study.

In conclusion, this integrated vision is extended into the clinical context, with a brief account of the insights offered by TTM to some problems of orthodox scientific practice.

THE HISTORICAL ORIGINS OF TRADITIONAL TIBETAN MEDICINE

Contemporary Tibetan doctors see their medical science as the flowing together of three great streams: the ancient medicine of Tibet itself, Indian medicine and Chinese medicine. It also contains elements from Persia, Mongolia and other lands. What follows is a historical sketch of TTM based mainly upon its founders and literature. The introduction and development of the various diagnostic and therapeutic components of TTM associated with each of these is too complex to be within the scope of this chapter.

The early history

What we know today as TTM emerged in Tibet during the seventh and eighth centuries CE. Before this, Tibetans had a medical and veterinary heritage based upon folk knowledge of the therapeutic qualities of local plants, salts, minerals and animal products. There had also been some significant visits from foreign doctors, such as the physicians sent from India by the Buddhist King Asoka (third century BCE), who unified India and spread medical science through Asia. Medical science is mentioned in various biographies of early regional kings, of note among whom are the fifth-century Lha-mtho-ri, who brought two eminent doctors from India to teach diagnostic procedures to Tibetans, and the sixth-century 'Bron-gnyan, whose son was successfully operated upon for cataracts, using a couching method with a golden scalpel.

In the first half of the seventh century, King Srong-btsan-sgam-po ruled over the first unified Tibet and a Tibetan empire. He brought civilization to his people by having scholars create an alphabet and grammar suited to the native tongue and by inviting scholars from the great civilisations of Asia. To introduce the best of medical science, he brought knowledge from India, China and Persia. This task was facilitated by the fact that his two main queens were the result of royal marriage alliances with China and Nepal. Of note during his reign were the translation of the *Great medical treatise* from Chinese and the transmission of knowledge from the Chinese master physician Han-wang-Hang, the Indian master physician Bharadhaja and the Persian master physician Galenos (which was probably a penname or nickname). These last three eminent doctors set down severally the essentials of their healing arts in texts in the new language. Moreover, they produced a seven-chapter treatise (*The weapon of the fearless*, which many scholars date as mid-seventh century, c. 660) based upon their mutual discussions and interaction. The first two physicians eventually returned to their homeland but Galenos remained as Court Physician, married and had three sons whom he trained as doctors and who subsequently spread the medical science in northern, central and southern Tibet. There was also a royal programme for training bright boys to become doctors, in which was established the first Tibetan medical school.

Box 4.1 details the scholarly tradition in TTM.

In the first half of the eighth century, many medical texts were translated into Tibetan (mostly from Chinese) and a first set of medical ethics were laid down for court and other physicians. During the latter half of the century, King

Box 4.1   The scholarly tradition in Tibetan medicine

Much of our current understanding of the history of Tibetan medicine is based on the widely held Tibetan traditional knowledge handed down through the generations and supported by much Tibetan written material dating from the eighth century onwards. Virtually all of the latter was destroyed during and after the Chinese occupation of 1959. Some facts are mentioned in Chinese court records of the seventh and eighth centuries. In general, Tibetans were excellent historians, maintaining written records of the activities of their monarchs and major scholars. This was particularly true from the eleventh century CE onwards. This generally accepted version of Tibet's medical history has been researched and documented on several occasions by the Wellcome Institute for the History of Medicine.

Khri-srong-lde-btsan (740–798 CE) firmly established Buddhism in Tibet. He was also determined to establish an excellent medical system and had eminent physicians from neighbouring lands translate various key medical texts of the great countries of Asia. Under his patronage, hundreds of bright children were also trained as translators. Of particular note was the work of the great translator Vairocana, who himself mastered and translated the fundamental texts of the Indian Buddhist medical system into a *Core treatise*, which was later to evolve into the famous *Fourfold treatise*, the foundation stone of the present Tibetan medical system. However, the main religious figure in Tibet at the time – Padmasambhava – judged it to be too early to introduce this system and decided to conceal the translations and instructions in a pillar of the great Samye monastery, to be discovered later when the time was right.

During this period a great wealth of contemporary Asian medicine came to Tibet. This king also had a considerable number of intelligent young men trained in the techniques embodied in these translations. Nine of them became most learned and were appointed Court Physicians. Of particular note was the first Gyu-thog yon-tan gon-po (pronounced Yutok Yeunten Gonpo), believed by Tibetans to have reincarnated some centuries later, as Yuthog the Second, to become the guardian and expounder of the Core treatise teachings concealed at Samye.

The ninth century saw a period of violent reaction to, and destruction of, the new wave of Buddhist and foreign culture introduced by King Khri-Srong. The empire crumbled and there was considerable anarchy. Some medical historians say that, although Buddhism suffered terribly, the medical tradition continued unaffected. This is doubtful (Skal-Bzang-Phrin-Las, 1997). Although much is recorded as having been translated, very few manuscripts remain from the early period. Whatever the case, this reactionary period halted the élan of development in medical science during some four short reigns but then triggered a vigorous revival of the intercourse with Indian medicine that was to continue for two centuries (Senior Staff of Tibetan Hospital 1990).

From the latter half of the tenth century, Tibetan medicine took its next significant step forward. Scholars of India and Tibet plied diligently between both lands, working hard to restore culture in Tibet and bring it the best that India had to offer. Known as *lotsawa*, or translators, these were not mere linguists but great minds, 'translating' in the very broadest sense the gems of one culture into another. From the tenth to the twelfth century, they not only restored Buddhism and medicine in Tibet but also considerably broadened their bases and firmly implanted a culture that was to last until the late twentieth century. Among other things, they translated one of the most important early medical texts, the *yan-lag brgyad-pa'i snying-po bsdus-pa* (*Quintessence of the eight branches of medicine*), in 120 chapters, along with its commentary, *Bza-ba'i 'od-zer* (*Moonbeams* c. 988).

The flowering of traditional Tibetan medicine

In the eleventh century, the most influential of the translators was Rin.chen-bzang.po (958–1055), who studied under 75 great Indian scholars and spent much time mastering the medical teachings of *Janadarna*, especially the 'Quintessence of the eight branches' text and its commentary. He taught, established and spread these medical teachings in Tibet. The lineages arising from his students considerably increased the practice of TTM. In all, over 150 texts were translated and edited under his guidance.

During this century, complex notions of the psychosomatic nature of the human being and his/her interdependence with the immediate and more distant universe were adopted, through the teachings of the *Kalachakra tantra*. Meyer (1981) describes this as the inheritance of: 'Indian concepts pertaining to the structure of the body, conception, physiology, pathology and therapy'.

History makes particular mention of nine master physicians of Rin.chen bzang.po's lineage towards the end of the eleventh century. Two of them brought new developments. A certain Shang-ston went to India and studied the 'Eightfold quintessence' extensively in Nalanda University under the great doctor Chadravi. He returned to Tibet with many teachings, which he translated. Another, Stod-ston, also went to India and studied these same works under Master Shintipa. Stod-ston is best known for instructing the Second Yuthog in the Moonbeams commentary on the Eightfold quintessence. During the last half of the century, Gter-ston-gra-pa-mngon-shes (1012–1090) discovered and revealed the Fourfold treatise hidden three centuries previously in the pillar of Samye monastery.

The twelfth century gave Tibet the most famous of its physicans – the Second Yuthog (1112–1203) – and the publication of its most famous medical work, the Fourfold treatise, which drew together in a masterly way all the elements that had entered Tibetan medicine up to that time. Much of subsequent TTM literature consists of commentaries to the Fourfold treatise.

The Second Yuthog is surrounded by legend and was doubtless an extraordinary figure who visited India many times and whose clear and broad mind was able to present an overview of all the various components present in the medical science of Tibet at the time. His work is the fruit of wide-ranging medical experience and considerable travel.

In the early to mid fifteenth century, two traditions of TTM, those of Byang and Zur, came to the fore (Box 4.2). Each was based upon the Fourfold treatise but held a different view as to its nature, had some slight differences of interpretation and some variance in plant recognition. The Byang and Zur systems, developed independently in the fifteenth century, cross-fertilized each other in the sixteenth century and virtually merged into one during the late seventeenth century, under the powerful influence of Regent sde-srid-sang-rgyas.

Box 4.2   The Byang and Zur systems of traditional Tibetan medicine

The *Byang* system originated with Jangdagpa (byang-bdag rnam-rgyal grags-bzang, 1395–1475). He and his followers composed many medical treatises, especially commentaries on the *Fourfold tantra*. Their system flourished in the north of Tibet. They held the *Fourfold treatise* to be a teaching given directly by the Buddha.

The *Zur* system started some fifty years later, in Southern Tibet, through Zurkhapa (zur-mkar mnyam-nyid rdo-rje, 1439–1475). A child prodigy, he was strongly influenced by the Yuthog Nyintik esoteric medical tradition stemming from the Second Yuthog. He dreamed that the extant versions of the *Fourfold treatise* and other related texts had become corrupted over the centuries, through additions and alterations, and that he should revise them. This he did meticulously, returning to Indian source documents and convening conferences of doctors from all parts of Tibet. His brief but important life gave a great renewal to TTM and launched one of its most famous traditions.

The fifth Dalai Lama (1617–1682) gained power over many Tibetan areas and became a powerful monarch. He founded several medical schools away from the new capital, Lhasa. His main disciple and future Regent, Desi Sangye (sde-srid-sangs-rgyas-rgya-mtsho, 1563–1705) was a brilliant scholar. Under his direction, a team of doctors and scholars studied the various commentaries of the Byang and Zur traditions on the Fourfold treatise and reported back to him on differences, discrepancies and moot points. From all this research, a major commentary, the *Blue vaidurya treatise*, was composed. The fifth Dalai Lama was not completely happy with his medical colleges and asked Desi Sangye to find a suitable location near Lhasa to found a new one. Thus the renowned Iron Hill (Icags-po-ri) Medical College was established. It was ordained that each monastery, in other words each district, would receive a doctor trained in this college. Thus it represented the beginnings of a public health system in Tibet. The political power of Desi Sangye's tradition – the Gelugpa school – at the time meant that this medical movement soon came to dominate medical practice in a great part of the Tibetan plateau. It effectively drew the Byang and Zur traditions into one and launched a new wave of TTM.

TRADITIONAL TIBETAN MEDICINE IN MODERN TIMES

In the eighteenth century, the Iron Hill Medical School became a model that was copied in eastern Tibet, at Kumbum in 1757, at Labrang in 1784, in Beijing at the Yonghegong around 1750 and also in Mongolia and Transbaikalia. There was a flowering of TTM in eastern Tibet during this century, under the influence of Dilmar Geshe, whose catalogue of materia medica became the widely accepted reference. Eastern Tibet is far less barren than central Tibet and is one of the main sources for many of the herbs, plants and trees used in TTM. Dilmar Geshe's famous disciple was the eighth Situpa, C Hoji Jungnay (chos-kyi byung-gnas, 1700–1774), a religious figure, grammarian, poet, scientist and doctor of great skills. He founded a medical school at Palpung, in the Tibetan kingdom of De-Ge in far-eastern Tibet, which was very receptive to the great wealth of classical Chinese knowledge of art, medicine and science.

Since the Chinese takeover in Tibet in the late 1950s and the mass exodus of many of its people, Tibetans in Tibet and across the world have struggled to maintain TTM. The main effort of preservation has been undertaken in Tibet itself. There, the practice of TTM has continued with Tibetans still relying on it for most medical interventions. At present, there are three major schools of Tibetan medicine where practitioners learn the art of TTM: one in Lhasa, one in the city of Zhiling in the province of Szechuan in China and a third university set up by the Tibetan government in exile in Dharmasala in Northern India. These schools take slightly different approaches to training, but essentially teach the same system. These schools continue to train practitioners of TTM to work in Tibet itself, Tibetan refugee centres in India and in other parts of the world. Practitioners of TTM have taken up residence in various Western countries and in some they are allowed to practice, albeit in a limited way.

RECENT DEVELOPMENTS IN THE UNITED KINGDOM AND IRELAND

There are practitioners of TTM scattered across various European countries, including the United Kingdom and Ireland. The first institute in these isles was inaugurated as the Tara Institute of Tibetan Medicine under the Tara Trust in Edinburgh in 1986. In the early 1990s the Institute began to invite esteemed practitioners and teachers of TTM from Lhasa, Zhiling and Dharmasala to the UK to teach TTM. The Tara Institute has provided a theoretical training in Tibetan medicine and has assisted Tibetan medical practitioners to come and live and practice in the UK and Ireland.

The Tara Institute has also fostered the development of a form of psychotherapy (Box 4.3).

> ## Box 4.3   The extension of traditional practice into modern times
>
> The Tara Institute of Tibetan Medicine has fostered the development of a form of psychotherapy called Tara Rokpa therapy. Akong Tulku Rinpoche, a Buddhist meditation master and former abbot of Drolma Lahang Monastery in Kham in eastern Tibet, has lived and worked in the UK since the mid-1960s. He is a Tibetan doctor by training and, although he has not practised the formal aspects of the herbal medicine, he has continued to practice the psychiatric, psychotherapeutic and psychological aspects. Akong Rinpoche's work has influenced the development of Tara Rokpa therapy, which is a form of psychotherapy that combines Eastern and Western understandings of the mind. This method in particular is bringing specialist aspects of TTM into a usable form for people living in the modern world. This Tara Rokpa therapy has been offered in many European countries, North America and Africa.

From its inception the Tara Institute has had a clear strategy to foster dialogue and exchange between conventional and complementary medical systems. As part of this strategy, the Institute has worked hard to ensure that TTM finds an appropriate place within the Western context. At all times it has emphasized safe practice and awareness of current understanding of medical problems within the West. The Institute has been clear about the need for exchange of understandings so that best practice might emerge. It continues to foster communication and dialogue between practitioners of each system and has encouraged Western patients and healthcare practitioners to discover the usefulness of TTM within the Western context. Part of this approach has been to introduce a 'herbal-only' form of TTM into the UK. This herbal-only form of TTM was devised by Mipam Rinpoche in the latter half of the nineteenth century and brought to the UK by Akong Tulku Rinpoche and other practitioners in the 1980s and 1990s. These herbal formulas are used by practitioners who work under the auspices of the Tara Institute and offer clinics in various cities including London, Edinburgh, Glasgow and Dundee and in the Scottish borders.

DEVELOPMENTS TOWARDS STATUTORY SELF-REGULATION

The community of practitioners of TTM has embraced the regulation of standards of training and practice of herbal medicine, including TTM, within the United Kingdom. Much of this work has been done under the aegis of the EHPA, with a strong emphasis on a thorough training of herbalists as one way of ensuring high standards of practice and safety for patients.

In the mid-1990s, the Department of Health began to discuss with the EHPA a possible move towards statutory self-regulation (SSR). This idea, though welcomed by those working in the field of Tibetan medicine, posed them some challenges. First, there was a need to set up an umbrella association that would represent TTM in all its aspects within the UK. At a meeting of practitioners of TTM in August 2002, hosted by the Tara Institute, it was agreed to set up and formally launch such an association. Thus the British Association of Traditional Tibetan Medicine (BATTM) was formed. It is now the official representative of TTM in the UK, although its full legal status is still to be finalized. The agreement to work together towards the common goal of SSR has held firm and is still the preferred approach of all involved in the Association. After its formation, the BATTM immediately endorsed the 'core curriculum', as developed by the EHPA, and, given the speed with which things were moving, began the work of finalizing a tradition-specific module on Tibetan herbal medicine, for inclusion in the 'core curriculum'.

In order to develop such a module, the practitioners based in the UK sought advice from the three universities who were already offering practitioner training (Lhasa, Dharmasala and Zhiling). These three universities have somewhat different approaches to training. It took time to agree an acceptable 'core'. There were also differences of understanding about the acceptable length of a course between the three universities in Asia, and between the UK model of higher education. A compromise was reached on this point by recognizing that, in the UK context, the training was focused clearly on the practice of medical herbalism. Further and higher training in other modalities of TTM could be offered at a later date, as postgraduate options. These other levels of training would be monitored through the new BATTM.

More recently, the Irish government has involved practitioners in a consultation process about the most appropriate way to regulate TTM in the Republic of Ireland.

As for the future, TTM through its umbrella organization BATTM is looking towards the European dimension. It intends to engage in professional communication and to participate in forming a European-wide association with its counterparts in Europe. BATTM is also aware that the United Kingdom has played a lead role in the drafting of the European Directive on Traditional Herbal Medicinal Products.

CONCLUSION

In conclusion, it is worth explaining one key feature of TTM. In this tradition, there has never been a split between the mind and body. Tibetan medicine has a very clear conceptual framework to understanding how the mind and body interact. Tibetan Buddhism, which is strongly influential on the system, emphasizes that cause and effect operate equally at both a mind and a body level. TTM has a clear theoretical exposition of the recursive interactions that occur between mind and body. The therapy emphasizes a multifactorial, or what it terms interdependent, understanding of phenomena and how they arise. This approach is used in understanding both the causation and the treatment of illness and equates well with the modern scientific view of Western medicine.

The key to understanding this system is the principle of 'the elements', both gross and subtle forces that influence one another across systemic boundaries, be they biological, psychological or social. An example would be the way outer elemental characteristics such as temperature can influence the body's constituents and have a causal role (albeit indirect) in the symptoms that a patient might experience. This systemic approach to all phenomena provides a rich source of understanding of human suffering in all its manifestations, with its strong emphasis on the non-separation of mind and body. Such a theoretical framework holds a promise of new approaches to mind/body medicine that are beginning to emerge in the Western context. TTM has theoretical and practical knowledge that has the potential to explain such phenomena as how the mind influences hormone and neurotransmitter release and regulation. It has developed within its system sophisticated methods for working directly with autonomic and endocrine functions. This opens out the promise of fruitful dialogue between TTM and the new mind sciences. Such possibilities were recently explored at the Second Congress of Tibetan Medicine held in Washington DC (2003), and are documented in a dialogue with the Dalai Lama (Goleman 2003).

TTM, in its modern form in Europe, has much to offer within the healthcare systems of modern society. It is because of a belief in such a 'fruitful dialogue' between traditional and modern clinical practice that practitioners in the UK and Ireland have chosen to work towards the achievement of SSR. From its earliest days, the development of TTM has been characterized by a willingness to borrow and to adapt, to interpret the understandings of others and to reinterpret them in the light of the Tibetan traditional 'ways of knowing'. Such borrowings and adaptations have been subject to scrutiny by scholarly practitioners, and to critical debate within communities of practice.

As TTM becomes more widely known and accepted in the countries of the West, it is expected that such an iterative development of knowledge will continue. The reciprocal extension of the knowledge base of herbal medicine, across all traditions, has a potential synergy of knowledge and understanding that could be of great benefit in the longer term.

References

Goleman D 2003 Destructive emotions (how can we overcome them), a scientific dialogue with Dalai Lama. Bantam, London

Meyer F 1981 Gso-ba rig-pa, le système médical tibétain. Editions du CNRS, Paris

Second International Congress of Tibetan Medicine: proceedings of the conference of 6–8 November 2003, Washington DC

Senior Staff of Tibetan Hospital (now the University College Hospital of Traditional Tibetan Medicine, Lhasa) 1990 Bod kyi gso rig pa, stod cha. In: Tibetan Medicine, volume 1. Tibetan People's Printing Press, Lhasa

Skal-Bzang-Phrin-Las 1997 Bod kyi gso rig byung 'phel gyi lo rgyus (The origin and development of Tibetan medicine). Chinese People's Tibetan Academic Press, Lhasa

Further reading

Alphen J V, Aris A, Meyer F et al 1995 Oriental medicine: an illustrated guide to the Asian arts of healing. Serindia Publications, London

Beckwith C 1979 The introduction of Greek medicine into Tibet in the seventh and eighth centuries. Journal of the American Oriental Society 99:297–313

Cordier P 1903 Introduction à l'étude des traités médicaux sanskrits inclus dans le Tanjur tibétain. Bulletin de l'Ecole Française d'Extrême Orient 3:604–629

Donden Y 1980 Health through balance, an introduction to Tibetan medicine. Snow Lion Publications, Ithaca

Emmerick R E 1977 Sources of the Rgyud-bzhi. In: Zeitschrift der Deutschen Morgenländischen Gesellschaft III, no 2 (suppl XIX. Deutscher Orientalistentag vom 28. September bis 4. Oktober 1975 in Freiburg im Breisgau)

Rechung Rinpoche J K 1973 Tibetan medicine. University of California Press, Berkeley

Thse Rnam K 2001 Gso-rig rgyud-bzhi'i 'grel-ba chen-mo. Chengdu, Sichuan Peoples' Publishing House

5

The development of integrated medicine with reference to the history of Ayurvedic medicine

Charles Cunningham

OVERVIEW

This chapter begins by describing the development of Ayurvedic medical practice, and by placing its historical development alongside that of other major systems of medicine that were mutually influential. It is therefore not appropriate to see Ayurvedic medicine as something that can be isolated from wider developments in knowledge.

There is then a short discussion of the theoretical principles of Ayurveda in terms of its relationship to both health and disease. Although Ayurveda needs to be seen in its own terms as a system of medicine, it is possible to draw some parallels with contemporary orthodox theories of health promotion. Indeed, such reconciling of core Ayurvedic constructs to other theories of medicine has been a feature of the way Ayurveda has developed historically.

In conclusion, the chapter briefly examines some safety issues around Ayurveda, particularly in interactions between Ayurvedic products and conventional medicine. It is argued that the traditional knowledge of toxicology, rooted in Ayurvedic scholarship, is as relevant to safe practice as any modern systems of quality control and licensing.

THE CONTEXT OF PRACTICE

The principles of Ayurveda are consistent with those of modern health promotion. They hold that health is essentially collective, the part being inextricably connected to the whole, and provide methods for raising the health of society as a whole at the same time as promoting individual health. Ayurveda describes health as the full expression of nature's intelligence at every level – mind, body, environment and cosmos – and this is reflected in its multiple therapeutic approaches. Ayurveda understands that subjectivity plays a central role in health – indeed it holds that the source of all order in physiology and in nature everywhere is consciousness itself. In common with modern health promotion, the Ayurvedic tradition emphasizes the necessity for integrating healthcare policy and practice with that of education, agriculture, transport, architecture and government.

It also shares with modern science a basis of empiricism. In common with all Vedic disciplines – yet in contrast with many types of folk medicine – Ayurveda is based upon empirical investigation and has always encouraged experimental verification (Pal 1989). Its ancient texts document argument and counterargument and the evaluation of alternative theories in the light of clinical experience (Sharma & Dash 1992):

"Every fact or observation has constantly been re-examined for a number of centuries."

(Dahanukar & Thatte 1989)

THE ORIGINS OF AYURVEDA

Ayurveda could well claim to be the world's oldest and most comprehensive system of medicine (Heyn 1987, Meulenbeld 1992).

Its exact origins are lost in the mists of antiquity but have been placed by scholars at around 6000 BCE. Even before any Ayurvedic documents existed, according to medical historian Henry Sigerist:

"an enormous amount of medical experience must have been gained empirically in the course of the centuries, and passed on orally from master to pupil ... Then the day came when somebody wrote down what he had learned, and the great compilations of Ayurveda took shape."

(Sigerist 1951, cited in Pal 1989)

The original Vedic text, *Rig Veda*, which appeared in written form for the first time around 2500 BCE, mentions surgical operations, prostheses and 67 medicinal plants. Even prior to this, archaeology reveals knowledge of public health issues. Facilities for public hygiene and sanitation, such as urban sewerage, fresh water supplies and numerous public-bathing houses are evident in archaeological sites in the Indus valley, such as Harappa and Mohenjo Daro, dating back to 3000 BCE.

The ancient medical text of Mesopotamia, *Codex hammurabi*, and that of Egypt, *Papyrus ebers*, are dated at 1700 and 1500 BCE respectively. These two medical texts are among the oldest that have survived to modern times.

The *Atharva Veda*, dated at 1200 BCE, documents herbal treatments for a hundred diseases and enumerates eight medical specialties: These are *Kayachikitsa* – internal medicine; *Shalya tantra* – surgery; *Shalakya tantra* – surgery of head and neck, opthalmology and otorhinolaryngology; *Vishagarvairodhika tantra* – toxicology; *Bhutavidya* – psychiatry; *Kaumarabhrutya* – gynaecology and paediatrics; *Rasayana tantra* – gerontology or the science of rejuvenation; and *Vijikarana tantra* – the science of fertility. There are a number of variant spellings of these specialties, but modern Ayurvedic practice continues to recognize the principles laid down in the *Atharva Veda*.

The prime emphasis of Ayurveda was always the promotion of health and prevention of disease; the need for surgery was regarded as the failure of prophylaxis. Nevertheless surgery was well advanced at an early date. Around the eighth and ninth centuries BCE, Dhanvantari and Atreya established two universities that persisted for centuries, providing training in surgical and medical specializations respectively. Shushrut, acknowledged as the originator of plastic surgery, elaborately describes in *Shushruta samhita*, a palm-leaf manuscript dated 500–300 BCE, the anatomy and pathology of the eye together with surgical procedures, for example for the removal of cataracts. His prognoses for various ocular diseases including glaucoma, together with his identification and treatment of both genetic and diet-induced diabetes mellitus, stand confirmed even today. Over a hundred surgical instruments are described in detail (Krishnamurthy 1991), as well as varied operations along with their preoperative and postoperative procedures. Shushrut is also accredited with describing the circulation of the blood, something only verified in detail by William Harvey in 1628. So, from the earliest times, practitioners of Ayurveda viewed it as a science that documented its theoretical and practical knowledge.

In the fourth and fifth centuries BCE, during which time Hippocrates gained fame in Greece, Ayurveda was systematically promulgated with the royal patronage of King Ashoka throughout the East, along with Buddhism. Medicinal herb gardens were established in each town. Medical historians, such as Castiglioni (1947), assert the 'priority of Indian to Hippocratic medicine', as discussed in Chapter 6 of this volume. Contemporary records are no longer available to inform us today about how such reciprocal learning happened. However, comparisons of the different herbal traditions indicate that there were interrelationships between them (see Chapter 6). The Encyclopaedia Americana (1849) states that: 'echoes of Indian classical medicine are traceable in the works of Hippocrates and Plato Timaens'.

In the first and second centuries CE, the Ayurvedic knowledge of plastic surgery spread to Arabia and Egypt. *Charaka Samhita*, the best-known work on Ayurveda, revised the earlier works of Atreya and Agnivesa. The medicinal use of metals was also described by Nagarjuna, who added to Sushrut's earlier work. This was the era that saw the growth of Greek and Roman medical systems with Dioscorides and Galen.

The following centuries saw the translation of Ayurvedic texts into Chinese. Travellers from China described Ayurvedic hospitals in India, sponsored by wealthy benefactors and known as 'houses of eternal bliss', dispensing free treatment to the poor of any country (Pal 1989). There are accounts of beautifully decorated purgatoria visited seasonally by the healthy. The works of Charaka and Shushrut were translated into Persian and Arabic, into Tibetan and thence other Asian languages, and perhaps into Greek. According to Sir William Hunter (Brook 1996), Arab medicine was founded on translations from these Sanskrit treatises. European medicine, down to the seventh century CE, was in turn based upon the Latin version of the Arab translation.

THE DEVELOPMENT OF AYURVEDA INTO THE PRESENT DAY

New texts continued to document the Ayurvedic materia medica, which included metals (*Dhanvantari Nighantu*), the preparation and combination of many more herbs and minerals (*Sharangadhara, Bhava Prakash*) and sexually transmitted diseases and their treatment (*Phirangaroga*). At this time in Europe, the practice of alchemy shifted through the Renaissance period to become the practice of medicine. Detailed knowledge of human anatomy became known through human dissection, something forbidden until this time in Christendom. Thus in different places, within different cultural traditions, the epistemology of medicine was being developed.

In the sixteenth and seventeenth centuries, the Muslims imposed Unani medicine in India. Later the British through the East India Company, on the one hand, transported knowledge of plastic surgery back to England and aroused academic interest in Ayurveda and, on the other, outlawed its practice in India in 1833. This was the time of Hahnemann's introduction of homeopathy and the discovery of anaesthetic gas in Europe.

In the nineteenth century, the rise in the West of germ theory, pasteurization and antisepsis revolutionized therapeutics and promised virtually to eradicate infections as causes of mortality. Many modern drugs, such as codeine, ephedrine, digitoxin, quinidine and caffeine, were derived from Ayurvedic plants. In the late nineteenth century, international interest in Ayurveda began. There was a concerted effort to restore Ayurveda and the industrial manufacture of Ayurvedic drugs started in different countries. As vaccination was utilized in Europe and the 'sulpha' drugs and streptomycin were developed, pharmaceutical companies began their analysis of thousands of Ayurvedic herbs for their biological actions.

It was in 1949, with the publication in the British Heart Journal of a report on the usefulness of the Ayurvedic herb *Rauwolfia serpentina* in the treatment of hypertension, that Ayurveda regained some of the status it had lost in the view of modern medicine. Reserpine was later isolated from this plant and its action (depletion of catecholamine stores) understood. Other such papers followed. The Indian Council for Medical Research began to coordinate systematic research into Ayurvedic flora and fauna, and the World Health Organization (WHO) began to promote collaborative international research into Ayurvedic herbal medicine.

The pharmacopoeia of Ayurveda is now known to comprise over 2000 medicinal herbs (Jain 1994) in more than 8000 combinations, documented in 70 or so ancient texts. Herbal medicine is just one of many therapeutic strategies that it employs.

AYURVEDA TODAY

Ayurveda was overshadowed by modern medicine for many reasons (Dahanukar & Thatte 1989). For a century, the Indian intelligentsia itself has embraced modern medicine, together with modern medicine's inherent scepticism and rejection of other systems, spurning their own Ayurvedic tradition.

Nevertheless, today the All India Ayurveda Congress represents over 300 000 physicians. In India, over 100 colleges grant a degree in Ayurveda after 5 years of study. There are 23 departments that award doctorates in Ayurvedic studies, and about 50 research institutes are engaged in research into Ayurveda (Zaman 1983). Nowhere is traditional medicine as integrated into the official health service as in India. Ayurveda in India cares for over 70% of the population, supported by more than 200 Ayurvedic hospitals and 14 000 dispensaries. Despite this, it has not been possible for foreigners to gain Ayurvedic training in India until recently (Welch 1995), and Ayurveda is only now becoming well known in the West.

Research in Ayurveda has been intense over the last 30 years, as is discussed further below. There has been a rapid growth in evidence for the efficacy of Ayurvedic therapeutics, an objective cited by Zaman (1983) as essential for integration of Ayurveda with modern medical practice. Much of this has focused on herbal remedies that have been tried and tested for centuries, for example in the treatment of diseases now known as cancer, cardiovascular disease, rheumatoid disease, asthma and other allergic disease, and viral diseases, particularly hepatitis A and B. For practitioners of Ayurveda, the documenting of the specialist knowledge base has been an important way of establishing rigour and gaining acceptability in the wider community of healthcare. That this strategy has been successful is evident in the integration of Ayurveda with scientific medicine in India.

An important characteristic of natural medicines is the presence of compounds that modulate, and in some cases are synergistic with, the compounds possessing major biological activity. The interrelationships of such compounds in plant materials is something that is easily missed by the reductionist approach of modern scientific methods, potentially leading to the dangerous side-effects of some synthetic drugs. The last 20 years have seen the standardization of raw materials and of manufacturing processes. There is a greater understanding of the principles of Ayurveda among practitioners of contemporary medicine, and the practice of Ayurveda is now more in accord with its foundational principles. Many associations around the world actively promote Ayurvedic education and publications, as well as herbal and mineral products.

Training in Ayurveda is offered by various organizations including the Institute of Naturopathy in Australia, the Ayurvedic Institute in New Mexico, and Maharishi Ayurveda (MAV) in India and other countries. It is anticipated that an accredited course leading to practitioner status will become available in the UK within the next 5 years, although currently practitioners train overseas.

In the UK today are many well-qualified Ayurvedic practitioners from India, as well as Western doctors who have trained in the discipline. Some have formed professional associations such as the Ayurvedic Medical Association (AMA) and the Maharishi Ayurveda Practitioners Association (MAPA). These are now working with practitioners of herbal medicine from other traditions to meet the government's requirement for self-regulation and ensure high standards of education, training and professional practice.

A personal account of the training of a contemporary Ayurvedic practitioner is given in Box 5.1.

Box 5.1 The professional formation of a contemporary Ayurvedic practitioner

As a medical student I learnt Transcendental Meditation (TM). At the time I did not realize it would profoundly influence my career. Over the next few years I experienced the benefits and met hundreds of TM meditators and heard how through TM they had been cured of illnesses from eczema to insomnia and from ulcers to migraine. There was obviously something significant going on.

In 1984 Maharishi, who had introduced TM, organized courses for doctors qualified in orthodox Western medicine on other strategies of healing from the same Vedic tradition. This he called 'Maharishi's Vedic Approach to Health'. It included Ayurveda. So for 18 months I studied in America and then at the postgraduate centre in the Ayurveda University in Jamnagar in Gujarat State, India.

One thing was very striking for all us doctors on this course. There is a certain style of thinking in which a doctor is trained. We noticed how in Ayurveda the exact same thinking was involved, but taken to new and exciting areas. Ayurveda is scientific in that it is systematic, logical and rational. However, the deductive processes therein could be applied not only to disease but also to understanding the cause of disease in particular individuals in terms of their nature, environment or lifestyle. It expands the thought processes beyond treatment to prevention and health promotion. Many of the strategies of healing are innate as opposed to external manipulations of drugs, surgery and radiation. The role of the physician as educator predominates and most of the healing is achieved by the patient using the new understanding imparted by the physician.

I have been practising Ayurveda over the past 19 years; it has been an inspiration. In general practice one is faced with up to 60 patients each day, most with about three or four problems. That is roughly 240 problems every day. But using Ayurveda the practitioner is focused on the health of the patients individually, and how to help them to enhance it. That is just one solution to all problems. The effect is to transform the experience of interaction with patients into a great joy, usually for both patient and doctor.

Dr Donn Brennan

THEORETICAL FOUNDATIONS OF AYURVEDA

Ayurveda speaks of the different levels *(koshas)* of the 'body' *(shirira)*, or of the illusion *(maya)* of the body that is actually nothing other than the display of pure energy or intelligence. The level of matter *(ana maya kosha)* is grosser than the level of energy *(prana maya kosha)*, which is grosser than the levels of mind *(mano maya kosha)*, then intellect *(buddhi maya kosha)*, bliss *(ananda maya kosha)*, and finally absolute intelligence *(sat chit ananda)*. Thus 'mind' denotes not only the more subjective aspect of the person but also a deeper level of organization present in the body. Box 5.2 offers a contemporary analogy for the Ayurvedic model of the human system.

Box 5.2 A modern metaphor for an ancient tradition

In order to understand the Ayurvedic model of the human system, it may be helpful to consider a contemporary analogy. The physical body is like the output from a computer system: it is constantly generated afresh and, contrary to superficial appearances, is the least stable component of the system. The software (operational instructions) is the biochemistry that runs on the hardware of the nervous system. Mental and subjective events are the programming that gives rise to biochemical messengers. Consciousness in its pure state – the experiencer, the essence of subjectivity, *veda* – is the programmer, the source of all intelligence within the system. Modifying the printout alone is no solution to faulty output; nor is piecemeal modification of the software: the programmer needs to be engaged to reprogram the system.

In clinical practice, it is most usual to use certain combinations of the five fundamental 'elements' (earth, water, fire, air and space) in the form of the three *'doshas'*. These roughly correspond to the subtle, functional energy level of the body – *prana maya kosha* – and are fundamental propensities within the physiology, as well as in the environment. The three *doshas* are known as *Vata*, *Pitta* and *Kapha*. Each of the three *doshas* has its characteristic site in the body and its own unique function. *Vata* is the tendency to move and expand (like air and space) and governs the functions of circulation, respiration, elimination, sexual reproduction, osmosis, neural conduction and creative thought. *Pitta* is the tendency to transform (like fire) and is responsible for digestion, metabolism, heat, energy and the critical faculty. *Kapha* is the tendency to cohere (like water and earth) and gives rise to the tissues and fluids of the body; it is associated with growth, strength, stability, beauty and affection. Equilibrium within and between the *doshas* is necessary for normal functioning of both mind and body.

Their role in pathogenesis and effective management constitute the *tridosha* theory, for which Ayurveda is best known.

Governed by the interaction of the *doshas*, the digestion and metabolic processes (*agnis*) transform food into the bodily tissues (*dhatus*), utilizing appropriate channels of transportation and communication (*shrotas*) and producing metabolic end products (*malas*). Ayurveda enumerates seven tissue types: plasma and interstitial fluid (*rasa*), blood corpuscles (*rakta*), muscle (*mamsa*), fat (*meda*), bone (*asthi*), bone marrow and nervous tissue (*majja*), and reproductive tissue (*shukra*). These make up the organs and organ systems just as they do in modern physiology. The *dhatus* form the basic structure of the body. Each of the seven has its own discrete function. *Mala* are metabolic end products that serve to support the functions of the body and are then excreted. The *tridosha* should be in a state of perfect equilibrium for the body to remain healthy.

Life (*ayuh*) is defined as:

"the conjunction of body, senses, mind and self (consciousness) and as synonymous with that which upholds and supports, that which animates and enlivens, that which goes on continuously."

(Sharma & Dash 1992)

Health (*swastha*) is defined as establishment in the Self (*veda*), equilibrium of *doshas*, *agnis*, *dhatus*, and *malas* together with soundness of senses, mind and soul (Dahanukar & Thatte 1989).

While attributing all illness to the loss of full expression of *Veda*, different 'causal' agents may be implicated at different levels. These include dullness of mind, imbalance of the *doshas*, weakening of the *agnis*, toxins in the *dhatus*, external agents, improper behaviour, etc. The same symptoms could have different causes in different people; and the same pathogenic factors could give rise to different disorders in different physiologies. Thus a skilled Ayurvedic physician is needed to make a correct diagnosis and this is done primarily through pulse diagnosis (*nadi vigyan*). Only when this is done can judicious preventive, dietary and behavioural measures be taken, or treatment prescribed for a disorder.

Six stages of pathogenesis are described, most of which precede the physical manifestations identified by modern diagnosis. These are accumulation, aggravation, dissemination, localization, manifestation and finally disruption. While prescribing measures to prevent illness from external pathogens, Ayurveda gives prime importance to the immunity (*bala*) of the host.

The reconciliation of Ayurvedic constructs, including the three *doshas*, with those of contemporary medicine has been attempted since the last century (Dahanukar & Thatte 1989, Wise 1845). The foundational principles of Ayurveda, together with an integration of them with modern scientific theory, has been offered by Maharishi Mahesh Yogi and is summarized by Wallace (1993). As we have seen above, this reconciliation of differing constructs is characteristic of an innate move to integration rooted in Ayurvedic principles. In India, this has facilitated the integration of traditional and modern medicine in the public system of healthcare. It is our hope that Ayurveda will, in the UK, be part of the contemporary move to more integrated systems of healthcare and medical practice.

SAFETY ISSUES

A small number of cases of adverse reactions between Ayurvedic and conventional medication have been well documented and researched (Fletcher & Aslam 1991, Thatte et al 1993). In some cases the mechanism of such inter-actions has been elucidated, but in other cases it remains obscure. Research is routinely performed into suspect cases by government-funded adverse drug reaction units in India. Such information, when known, can obviously be included on all packaging and instructions to patients, doctors and dispensers of such products. Fortunately, however, cases of adverse side-effects appear to be exceptional.

Toxicology is a well-developed specialization of Ayurveda with elaborate, painstaking and proven procedures for detoxifying poisonous but potentially therapeutic herbs and metals (Thatte et al 1993). However, with the burgeoning of demand around the world for alternative medicines, and because of aggres-sive marketing, traditional instructions for 'over-the-counter' (OTC) medications have been neglected. Such instructions include dosage, time of day, relation to mealtime, diet, and '*anupanam*' or a substance to be taken with the medication to facilitate its assimilation. With recent improvements in regulation, however, measures have been taken to ensure that high standards of quality control and licensing, already operated by the more professional organizations, are made universal for all Ayurvedic medicines. It is through an adherence to the rigour of traditional knowledge that patients can be kept safe in modern times.

It is critical that the modern practitioners pay as much attention to traditional prescription instructions as to modern manufacturing quality assurance processes. By combining ancient ways of knowing with modern systems of regulation, Ayurveda is in a position to make a major contribution to world health, and to healthcare in Britain.

CONCLUSION

This brief account of the history and development of Ayurveda has emphasized its compatibility with other systems of medicine, as evidenced today in the way

Ayurvedic medical practice is fully integrated into the care of patients in India. There has always been a scholarly tradition in relation to Ayurvedic practice, with written texts surviving from the earliest times. It is thus possible to trace how it has developed in interaction with medical traditions elsewhere in the world. This influence can be documented from the earliest times, and is part of the implicit philosophy of the practice.

Because of this implicit orientation to integration, perhaps more than at any other time in it its long and venerated history, Ayurveda is poised to be a major influence on the worldwide move towards integrated medicine more generally.

References

Brook C H 1996 Calendar of the correspondence of Dr William Hunter 1740–1783. Wellcome Unit for the History of Medicine, Cambridge

Castiglioni A 1947 (translated Krumbhaar E B) A history of medicine. Alfred A Knoff, New York

Dahanukar S A, Thatte U M 1989 Ayurveda revisited: Ayurveda in the light of contemporary medicine. Popular Prakashan, Bombay

Encyclopædia Americana 1849 Lea & Blanchard, Philadelphia

Fletcher J, Aslam M 1991 Possible dangers of Ayurvedic herbal remedies. Pharmacological Journal 247(6656):456

Heyn B 1987 Ayurvedic medicine. Thorsons, Wellingborough

Jain S K 1994 Ethnobotany and research on medicinal plants in India [review]. Ciba Foundation Symposium 185:153–164; discussion 164–168

Krishnamurthy K H 1991 A source book of Indian medicine: an anthology. BR Publishing, Delhi

Meulenbeld G J 1992 The many faces of Ayurveda. Ancient Science Life 11(3–4):106–113

Pal M N 1989 Ayurveda: an international overview – part I. Ancient Science Life VIII(3/4):235–240

Sharma R K, Dash V B 1992 Agnivesha's Caraka Samhita. Chowkhamba Press, New Delhi

Sigerist H E 1951 A history of medicine. Oxford University Press, Oxford

Thatte U M, Rege N N, Phatak S D et al 1993 The flip side of Ayurveda. Journal of Postgraduate Medicine 39(4):179–182, 182a–182b

Wallace R K 1993 The physiology of consciousness. MIU Press, Iowa

Welch C 1995 Studying Ayurveda in India. Ayurveda News 4.1:9

Wise T A 1845 Commentary on the Hindu system of medicine. Medical Services, Bengal

Zaman H 1983 A profile of traditional practices in the South-East Asia region. In: Bannerman R et al (eds) Traditional medicine and health care coverage. WHO, Geneva

Western herbal medicine – gender, culture and orthodoxy

6

Peter Jackson-Main (with a contribution by Julie Cox)

OVERVIEW

This chapter explores Western herbal medicine, from its origins to its place in contemporary society. It argues that Western herbal medicine cannot be seen as solely the product of a geographic location. Rather, the practice represents a synthesis of different ways of knowing, located in cultural understandings that transcend geopolitical boundaries.

In the discussion, it is argued that the history of herbal medicine in Europe has to be read from a gendered perspective. The association of herbal practice with women herbalists led to its decline from the fourteenth century. It is only with the re-emergence of women in orthodox healthcare professions that herbal medicine has regained formal recognition.

In the conclusion, the question of professional identity is explored at the present historical moment. It is suggested that the movement to statutory self-regulation may pose threats as well as opportunities to the community of practitioners. It is through a shared set of values that the contemporary herbalist community will defend and extend its traditional practice.

THE NATURE OF WESTERN HERBAL MEDICINE

The term 'Western herbal medicine' could itself be somewhat misleading. It is currently employed to refer to the usage of medicinal plants that have been indigenous to Europe, North America and Australia, as opposed to older systems, such as Ayurveda, Tibetan medicine and Chinese herbal medicine, with which it now coexists in these areas. These latter disciplines are fenced off by virtue of having evolved in an unbroken line within strict geographical boundaries; they are defined not only by their methods and philosophy, but also by their place of origin, no matter that they have been transplanted into foreign soil.

By contrast, Western herbal medicine cannot really be thus segregated. It crosses many national and cultural boundaries, often making free use of plants that are, or were, the specific materia medica of older traditions such as Ayurveda and Chinese herbal medicine. It draws, some would say borrows, philosophical premises from its older siblings, and it has developed its own in addition. Within its boundaries, if indeed it admits of such, are found traditional healers working from an understanding of esoteric and energetic models, alongside modern *phytotherapists* following a more strictly biomedical premise. It is therefore nothing if not a broad church, and one that almost defies definition.

It has often been popularly assumed that Western herbalists are little more than ersatz doctors who prescribe herbal remedies rather than pharmaceutical drugs. The oft-quoted fact that many modern pharmaceutical drugs started life as plants has led to a situation where herbs themselves are frequently thought of as being nature's counterpart to the refined and specialized materials produced by the pharmacist, the idea that there is 'a herb for every ailment' being essentially no different from 'a pill for every ill'. Indeed, in the marketplace, there has been a tendency, until growing pressure from legislative bodies has curbed this, to present herbal medicines as alternatives to drug medicines. This presupposes that one might simply substitute like for like, the particular malady or symptom being the defining reason for choosing the remedy.

This emphasis has been reflected in the high street in the UK, with single plants such as St John's wort and echinacea becoming prominent and well known to buyers as remedies. Qualified herbalists, on the other hand, would more usually work with *polypharmacy*, the combining of several plants in the same formula. Knowledge and understanding of the synergistic effects of herbs placed together is one of the considerations that sets herbal practice apart from the commercial focus of over-the-counter (OTC) herbal remedies. Recently proposed European legislation in the form of the Directive on Traditional Herbal Medicinal Products (DTHMP 2004), together with the statutory registration of herbal practitioners, will henceforth govern the safe sale of OTC remedies and encourage the sale and use of old and trusted formulas, perhaps enabling us to preserve Europe's rich heritage in this respect.

Popular misconceptions about herbal medicine has tended to mask the real truth, which is that Western herbalists, by and large, are more interested in people than they are in diseases. Thus, the underlying rationale for delivering a specific treatment must have at least as much to do with the individual who is to receive it as it does with the name of the presenting condition. In this respect herbal practitioners in the Western tradition are the true descendents of Hippocratic medicine, which focused attention on the patient rather than the disease and regarded the body as a whole rather than a series of parts, in contrast to modern medics who invoke the Hippocratic Oath, yet whose philosophy and methodology is actually a world apart.

One of the crucial differences between the Greco-Roman tradition evident in the works of Hippocrates and modern medical theory lies in the latter's emphasis upon pathology rather than process. In the Hippocratic model, the pathway to disease, or imbalance, lay in the lifestyle choices of the individual who, by making adjustments in diet ('Let thy food be thy medicine and thy medicine thy food') and committing to certain corrective practices, could reverse the trend towards illness and thus re-establish health. By contrast, the disease-oriented approach of the modern medical profession at large is still evident in the thrust of research that concentrates upon targeting and 'curing' specific diseases. Modern medicine has been notoriously resistant to the notion that one might better one's condition by reforming one's diet, lifestyle and so forth – an idea that is fundamental to systems that emphasize balance and correction as the keys to restoring health.

It is problematic that these underlying dynamics have, even for the modern Western herbalist, been largely submerged in the contemporary preoccupation with scientific reductionism, in the quest for active constituents and physiological pathways, and in the search for empirical evidence. For, whilst the scientific scrutiny of herbal medicines has yielded much of value, it has done little or nothing to shed light upon the true role of the herbalist. It is my contention that the herbalist owes more to these much older, traditional ideas than to the newer rationales that have been introduced in modern times. Furthermore, it is in relation to methods of practice, underlined by such philosophical understandings, that the modern conceptualization of the professional Western herbalist is derived.

It may be true that some, concerned about such a professional model, and lacking the secure foundations of a coherent traditional system (such as Ayurveda or Traditional Chinese Medicine) have all but turned their backs upon the traditional strands in Western herbal medicine, taking refuge in the evidence base of modern, 'rational phytotherapy'. But how has this happened? One has only to look at the unfortunate classification of Ayurveda and TCM in group III in the House of Lords Select Committee report (2000), alongside other systems of healing for which there exists 'no credible evidence base', to understand why practitioners would be concerned at all costs to avoid such stigmatization. As may be seen elsewhere in this book, this development has been much influenced by previous skirmishes with the orthodoxy.

The House of Lords' Select Committee report (2000) itself brings a couple of considerations into view. First, the placing of Western herbal medicine in category I, whilst seeming to give it the accolade of respectability and scientific veracity, has done the *practice* of herbal medicine no real favours. It validates those manufacturing and supplying remedies, presenting their wares as credible and proven; however, it does not in any way honour the truth of Western herbal practice in its holistic and traditional aspects, particularly in segregating it from its sister 'ethnic' traditions.

Secondly the report, in appearing to relegate whole systems of medicine to something approaching a ghetto, opens itself up to the charge of failing to give a proper account of that which it cannot understand. There we must simply agree to differ with the authors of the report. It is at least an honest statement of opinion. There is little in orthodox Western science that resonates in any way with any of the traditional systems of medicine that have prevailed upon this planet from time immemorial. That is equally true of Western herbal medicine, at least as far as its traditional roots and origins go.

THE ORIGINS OF WESTERN HERBAL MEDICINE

The origins of what we now call Western herbal medicine can be traced to a few diverse geographical and historical locations:

- the ancient Greco-Roman world
- the pre-existing indigenous practices of the British Isles and of Europe
- the New World opened up by the European explorers.

The Greco-Roman origins of European herbal medicine

The first of these strands is traceable back to around 1250 BCE with the Egyptian-born Greek physician Asclepius. Egypt and Mesopotamia were already known for a strong healing tradition in which herbal medicines played a significant part, with manuscripts dating back to 2500 BCE. It is likely that some of this knowledge itself had been taken from the Hindu *Rig Veda* (2500 BCE), which, in its later versions, lists over 1000 herbs in a medicinal context.

Thus, there may well indeed be an ancient connection between one of the most long-standing and venerable natural healing traditions of the world, Ayurveda, and what later developed in Europe (see Chapter 5). The ancient Middle Eastern, Arabian or Greco-Roman healing tradition Unani Tibb is a significant bridge between the two systems that survives to this day, and whose influence can also clearly be seen in medieval European (Galenic) medical practice.

Hippocrates (460–377 BCE) would have inherited the same tradition, and with his advent came the formulation of a Western style of medicine based upon plant remedies, yet introducing a more systematic rationale for diagnosis and pathogenesis. This rational tradition was expanded by the Greek physician and philosopher Galen (130–200 CE), whose theory and practice continued in popularity in Europe up to the seventeenth century.

However, the first comprehensive herbal in this tradition was compiled by Dioscorides, a Greek physician and doctor to the Roman army in the first century CE. His work, *De materia medica*, owed much to Hippocrates, but expanded the pharmacopoeia to include descriptions of over 600 herbs, many of them still in use today. *De materia medica* continued in use as a reference work in herbal pharmacology for almost a millennium, although it was not translated into English until 1933, by John Goodyer.

Throughout the Dark Ages in Europe and the British Isles, 'official' medicine was largely kept alive in the monasteries, which were the chief guardians and repositories of academic activity until the tenth century, and where monks were responsible for continuing to study and translate medical texts. However, as we shall see, other practitioners, largely unrecorded, were almost undoubtedly operating at the same time.

The enrichment of the European herbal tradition from further abroad was first evident in the fourteenth century, when explorers began to open up trade routes with India and China, and then in the fifteenth century, the New World was discovered. The subsequent appearance of spices, mainly used in culinary art, was also accompanied by that of new medicinal plants, and with the invention of the printing press in the fifteenth century the first popular herbals began to appear.

One of the most famous herbals was that of the London surgeon and botanist John Gerard, which was published in 1597. Although his *Herball* was a reworking of older texts, it was also imbued with his own very considerable experience both as a practitioner and as a horticulturalist with a strong interest in plants from all over the world (Woodward 1985).

It was Nicholas Culpeper, however, whose name became almost synonymous with herbal medicine, and remains so to this day. Culpeper, although himself from a privileged background, was something of a revolutionary and a champion of the common man; indeed he was known as 'the people's herbalist' His avowed desire was to break the monopoly of the Royal College of Physicians and make medicine accessible to the less fortunate by birth and circumstance. This he attempted to do by translating the *London pharmacopoeia* from Latin into English, much to the fury of the orthodoxy. His main work, *The complete herbal,* was published in 1649, and his insistence upon using the English names for plants, rather than the Latin that had been universal up till that time, rendered his book one of the most popular and accessible herbals of all time, with over 40 editions having been published up to the present day: indeed, it has never been out of print (Culpeper 1995).

Culpeper was a firm adherent to the 'Doctrine of Signatures', which dated back to the Swiss physician and alchemist Paracelsus in the previous century. The 'Doctrine of Signatures' provided a system for classifying herbal remedies according to affinities to organs suggested by the colour and shape of the plant: yellow for the liver, for example, or red for blood. Although this system was widely misunderstood, and so eventually devalued, it is difficult to get away entirely from some of the obvious correlations: just think of dandelions (yellow flowers – liver remedy) or hawthorn (red berries – heart and circulation).

Indigenous healers and the witch craze

It is self-evident that, whilst all the academic development was in progress, herbal medicine was popularly practised according to indigenous oral traditions that have largely escaped record. In this connection we have to consider that the official history of herbal medicine, as of so much else, is male dominated. However, it is the role of women that interests us particularly as we enter this lesser known domain.

"although in its original mode herbal medicine was most probably practised in local communities, largely by women, this is barely reflected in contemporary accounts."

(Mills & Bone 1999)

In the period of feudalism following the Norman invasion of Britain (1066 CE), women were excluded from taking any major office in the community, from pursuing specialist occupations or crafts, and were also rarely able to hold any land in their own right (Goldberg 1997, Middleton 1981). They were therefore largely powerless in political terms, and had no legal identity of their own (Box 6.1).

Box 6.1   The role of women in feudal Britain

Women's sphere of power was limited to the household (Middleton 1979). The feudal mode of life needed a constant supply of labour and a married woman's fertility and her work in bringing up children was her best asset. Being located in the household also allowed women to pursue tasks such as brewing, making cloth, hay and grain, as well as taking care of poultry, dairy cattle and doing craft work. From an early age, children would help in this work, rather than being a burden to their mothers. In their role taking care of children and men, women were also responsible for the family's health and, located within the household, were in a position to grow herbs that were a vital element of health provision in feudal times.

Healing under the feudal system was therefore based in the domestic domain and linked to the role of women in the family. Society was largely patriarchal in the feudal system, stretching down in authority from God to the king, to the lord of the manor and then to the male head of household. With no access to power in the church or in wider mediaeval society, women's roles in household production and as cooks, housekeepers, nurses and midwives allowed them to counter their lack of power elsewhere. As midwives, women presided over life and death at childbirth and they also had key roles in fertility, impotence and death.

In the fourteenth century feudal society came under great stress owing to the numbers of people who died from the Black Death (Gottfried 1983). Labour systems broke down when there were not enough peasants to work the demesnes. Even the lords and clergy could not survive infection. There was a loss of control in patriarchal society and social structures became insecure, as did the individuals who lived in that society. Individuals turned on their masters and there was widespread social unrest, but they also turned on women healers whose role was linked to pagan rituals and magic. A study of the witch craze in South West Germany showed that midwives were one of the most likely categories to be accused of witchcraft.

Women healers used herbs to heal members of their family, neighbours in the community and to assist in the rituals of birth and death. They also used herbs for many other purposes, such as driving out demons. A herb such as potentilla might be used to drive out the demon of fever, already blurring the distinction between healing and witchcraft. But this was further confused when the same herb would also be used to drive out witches. Herbs were also used in the rites of witchcraft. They were woven in with superstition, local customs and practices. Herbs such as cumin, basil and vervain could be used to make love potions that might be commissioned by local lovesick villagers in the community. Herbs might also be used to divine the future, while tansy, honesty, garlic and St. John's wort were used to ward off the evil eye or keep elves, goblins and spirits at bay.

Women would not necessarily see themselves as witches, but their extensive use of herbs and the blurring of distinctions between healing and magic meant that this might be how others saw them. Pre-Christian religion and local superstition might be called upon to bring good luck to individuals or to the community as a whole. Some women seen as witches might put a hex on others to cause sickness or harm livestock. The equating of superstition and magic with the use of healing herbs was all bound up with the complex role of women and may even have consequences for the way herbal medicine is perceived today. Both before and after the witch craze, the powerful concept of the 'wise woman' who could be called for to deliver babies or abate fevers was well known.

However, those who were perceived to have 'magic powers' might also find themselves being blamed for catastrophes and misfortunes, such as crop failures, the sudden death of livestock, or indeed, the Black Death itself. In this context it was perhaps a mixed blessing that women survived the plague up to six hundred times better than men (Russell 1980).

By the late fifteenth century, witchcraft had come to be seen as a very real threat to religious orthodoxy. Witches were firstly seen as pagans and later as devil worshippers (MacDonald 1991). The craze was most severe where there was social tension, plague and famine. Ninety per cent of those tortured and killed for being witches in England were women (Russell 1980). Although men were also killed, these were often husbands of women who had been accused, and were seen as having been contaminated by their wives (Trevor-Roper 1978).

By the seventeenth century, healthcare came to be viewed more as a valid and valued profession in the world outside the extended household. Herbals were written (Dumfermline District Libraries 1980). Physiomedical and Eclectic schools of herbal medicine, among others, sprang up. Theories of the practice of herbal medicine were debated, based initially on research into traditional herbal practice.

By the late eighteenth century witchcraft no longer existed. Science, liberalization of religion and a move from personal to institutional ties helped to create a different worldview. Medicine and healing became professions, part of that new rational society, but now falling into the domain of men. Medicine as a profession, whether orthodox or alternative and complementary, was not to be practised by women again in any significant numbers until the twentieth century.

"Our great-great-grandmothers are back. They may be wearing white laboratory smocks and using main-frame computers, but our great-great-grandmothers are indeed back."

(Mills & Bone 1999)

The coming of age of Western herbal medicine

The history recounted so far may paint a rather bleak picture of the state of Western herbal medicine as it moved into the nineteenth century. Brutally separated from its grass-roots traditional origins, infiltrated and commandeered by male-dominated oligarchies, forced to surrender to the rational and empirical values of the scientific medical world, herbal medicine in the UK at the end of the eighteenth century was beleaguered to say the least. This started to change in the mid-nineteenth century.

In the early part of the century, Albert Coffin, an English medical doctor, went to America and was successfully treated for tuberculosis by a Native American woman healer after conventional medicine had failed to restore him. Subsequently he met Dr Samuel Thompson, the American medical reformer and founder of the Physiomedical school, who imparted the techniques of physiomedicalism to him (Box 6.2).

Box 6.2 The Physiomedicalists and the Eclectics

Physiomedicalism was based largely upon the practices of the Native Americans, gathered by the early pioneers as they moved through the continent. It was based upon the idea that what was necessary to heal the human body was to stimulate its own powers of self-defense and self-regeneration (Coffin 1856). It also made use of naturopathic techniques such as hydrotherapy and dietary reform. Thompsonian herbalism, still taught in some schools today, was to become a keystone of herbal practice both in the USA and in Britain.

Closely allied to the Physiomedicalists were the Eclectics. As the name suggests, these were healers who selected elements from various different systems, including the native knowledge of the American Indians. Their materia medica was also almost entirely herbal, and they were famous for their success in treating chronic degenerative conditions that defeated the orthodox medics. One of their number, Dr John Christopher, was to reintroduce this style of herbalism to the UK when he came to establish a Master Herbalist diploma here in 1982.

Dr Coffin arrived back in England in 1839 and began to lecture on the practices and remedies he had learnt in America. However, he was met with hostility and indifference, and so he decided to espouse herbal medicine and work for the preservation of the knowledge he had acquired. Thus, with a select community of sympathetic doctors and lay practitioners, he was instrumental in founding the National Association of Medical Herbalists, later to become the National Institute of Medical Herbalists (NIMH).

Even today, the Western herbalist's materia medica still contains many plants that were originally exclusive to North America – for example, echinacea, black cohosh, golden seal and partridge berry. This is a testimony to the profound influence of Physiomedical and Eclectic herbalism on today's practitioners.

The nineteenth century was extremely important for the consolidation of orthodox or 'mainstream' medicine. The three major classes of medical practitioners – the physicians, the apothecaries and the surgeons – were organizing to fence off their professional domains and preclude lay and non-medical practitioners. Universities were increasingly the repositories and disseminators of medical know-how. The rapidly developing orthodoxy was keen to lay claim to exclusivity over both remedies and methods, and based itself squarely upon the emerging scientific rationales. Such manifestations of professional behaviours for protectionist or defensive purposes are discussed in Chapter 1.

The degree to which herbal practitioners had been marginalized was clearly demonstrated in legislative developments in the early to mid-twentieth century (Griggs 1997). In their continuing quest for recognition, the herbalists tabled a bill in Parliament in 1923, which was supported by over 130 MPs. However, the government did not grant time for the bill to go further, and it was dropped.

After the war, Bevan, who was Minister for Health at the time, offered herbalists a chance to work in the newly founded NHS, but only as poorly paid subordinates to the medical profession. The herbalists chose to remain outside the system.

It was not until the drafting of the Medicines Act 1968 that the herbalists succeeded in enacting in statutory legislation the right to practice herbal medicine and dispense herbal remedies. This significant campaign was coordinated by the late Frederick Fletcher Hyde, one-time president of the NIMH and of the British Herbal Medicine Association (BHMA). He saw that, unless action was taken, herbal medicine would have been finally and formally outlawed in the UK by the 1968 Act. The clauses that he was responsible for introducing into the Act, notably Sections 12:1 and 12:2, still underpin the legal basis for the practice of herbal medicine in the UK today (see also Chapter 9).

In this respect herbal practitioners in the Western tradition are the true descendents of Hippocratic medicine, which focused attention on the patient rather than the disease and regarded the body as a whole rather than a series of parts, in contrast to modern medics who invoke the Hippocratic Oath, yet whose philosophy and methodology is actually a world apart.

WESTERN HERBAL MEDICINE IN CURRENT TIMES

In the latter part of the twentieth century there was a proliferation of interest in herbal medicine in the UK, as across the Western world generally. This was probably fed by a growing measure of disenchantment with the mainstream medical option, and a desire on the part of a significant minority to return to traditional values enshrined in ancient systems. The spiritual renaissance of the 1960s was the harbinger of an explosion in opportunities to experience these modalities first hand. Traditional practitioners from China and India, in particular, found uniquely in the UK an environment that both welcomed and supported them. Such traditional practices included herbal medicine, yoga, meditation, massage, acupuncture and other forms of holistic healthcare.

Increased globalization also made new plant remedies accessible to the public, and to the practitioner. As we have seen, this was nothing new, as interest in exotic plants dates back to the fourteenth century, and from the nineteenth century the practice of herbal medicine owed a great deal to plants imported from America. However, with the advent of scientific research into plants, both on the part of the pharmaceutical industry and by herbal interests, plants that for centuries had been the stock-in-trade of Chinese medicine or Ayurveda began to pass into regular usage by Western practitioners. Examples here include dong quai (*Angelica sinensis*), ashwaghanda (*Withania somnifera*), ginseng (*Panax quinquefolium*) and ephedra (*Ephedra sinica*).

Other botanical remedies were forthcoming from areas such as the Amazon basin and South America. In the former Soviet Union, research into the biomedical aspects of plant medicine was part of applied mainstream science. The use of Siberian ginseng (*Eleutherococcus senticosus*) as an aid to building stamina in athletes, gymnasts and cosmonauts is one example of the application of traditional knowledge to modern life.

Such newly discovered plants have now become well established in the Western materia medica. Although some from the ethnic traditions have criticized this as an uninformed and possibly illegitimate usage, there is no doubt that many Western practitioners hold them in high esteem for the benefits they bring.

Nevertheless, among the practitioner community there is still a concern that the practice of herbal medicine may be distancing itself from its roots. In its traditional context, herbal medicine would have been a local indigenous practice. In the age of the 'global village' it could be argued that the local context has been expanded to include the whole planet. However, common sense argues that self-sufficiency in medicine, as in food and other resources, is best served by thorough knowledge and intelligent use of the resources of one's immediate environment – 'we must learn to live under our own fig tree':

"the best healing plants and foods come from our own backyards. To till the soil, plant the seeds, put in fruit trees, and let the medicinal 'weeds' thrive in our own yards, picking them at just the right time for each, enjoying the sun and wind and rain ... "

(Christopher & Gileadi 1987)

CONCLUSION

By defining herbal medicine as a graduate entry profession, there is a danger that the emphasis on academic learning may eclipse traditional values and practices. The introduction and consolidation of herbal medicine in universities is a vital step in the fight for recognition, and a coming of age of Western herbal medicine. At the same time, it echoes the process of exclusive professionalization that characterized the medical profession's assault on the lay community of practitioners in the nineteenth century. As Christopher Hobbs, the well-known American herbalist and botanist, recently observed to a close colleague of mine, 'Let's not forget that some of the greatest herbalists have come out of apprenticeships'. Furthermore, there has to be a place still for respected local healers/herbalists, with their backyard plants (organically grown or collected from wild sustainable sources), and the lore that has infused the practice of herbal medicine from time immemorial. And as Dr John Christopher was fond of saying, we should have 'a herbalist in every home, a practitioner in every community' (Christopher, 1993).

This vision is something that herbal practitioners I know from many different walks and traditions still hold in their hearts. With a nod also to the philosophical and sociopolitical example of Nicholas Culpeper, it places emphasis upon the ubiquity and accessibility of plant medicines, and upon the role of ordinary people using traditional knowledge in order to maintain health. It is, in my view, an essential counterpoint to the considerations of professionalization and the creation of an orthodoxy.

References

Christopher J 1993 A legacy of courage. Christopher Publications, Springville, Utah

Christopher J, Gileadi C 1987 Every woman's herbal. Christopher Publications, Springville, Utah

Coffin A 1856 A botanic guide to health and the natural pathology of disease. British Medico-Botanic Establishment, London

Culpeper N 1995 Culpeper's complete herbal: a book of natural remedies for ancient ills. Wordsworth Editions, Ware

DTHMP 2004 The traditional herbal medicinal products directive, 2004/24/EC. Official Journal of the European Union, 30 April

Dunfermline District Libraries 1980 The 17th century witch craze in West Fife: a guide to the printed sources. Dunfermline District Libraries, Dunfermline

Goldberg P J P 1997 Women in medieval English society. Sutton, Stroud

Gottfried R S 1983 The Black Death: natural and human disaster in medieval Europe. Hale, London

Griggs B 1997 The new green pharmacy: the story of Western herbal medicine. Vermilion, London

House of Lords' Select Committee on Science and Technology 2000 Complementary and alternative medicine, 6th report. Stationery Office, London

MacDonald M 1991 Witchcraft and hysteria in Elizabethan London. Tavistock/Routledge, London

Middleton C 1979 The sexual division of labour in feudal England. New Left Review 113:147–168

Middleton C 1981 Peasants, patriarchy and the feudal mode of production in England: feudal lords and the subordination of peasant women. Sociological Review 29:137–154

Mills S, Bone K 1999 The principles and practice of phytotherapy. Churchill Livingstone, London

Russell J B 1980 A history of witchcraft, sorcerers, heretics and pagans. Thames & Hudson, London

Trevor-Roper H 1978 The European witchcraze of the 16th and 17th centuries. Penguin, Harmondsworth

Woodward M 1985 Gerard's herbal. Bracken Books, London

7

The relationship of classical Greek medicine to contemporary Western herbalism:

an exploration of the idea of 'holism'

Victoria Pitman

OVERVIEW

The focus of this chapter is an examination of some of the original Greek sources that explicate the philosophical thinking embodied and embedded in the practice of the ancient Greek doctors. The chapter argues that the philosophy influenced all that a physician did. Further, it is suggested that a careful reading of the Hippocratic corpus uncovers a conceptualization of 'holism' that is still found today among contemporary practitioners.

The chapter therefore questions the perceived lack of connection in Western herbalism to its historical roots. This seems to contrast with Chinese, Ayurveda and Tibetan traditional medicine (see Chapters 3–5). The chapter concludes by suggesting that further research is needed both into the historical origins of Western herbal medicine, and also into the interrelationships with other great medical systems such as Ayurveda (Pitman 2004). Such research, as well as being of interest to historians and philosophers of medicine, offers important insights to problems of diagnosis and therapeutic strategies for the modern practitioner.

BACKGROUND

This chapter reports the results of an investigation into sources of holism in ancient Greek medical theory and practice as found in the Hippocratic corpus. The corpus is the surviving record of the ideas and practices of physicians of the fifth and fourth centuries BCE, which deeply influenced Galen and became the foundation for the Western medical tradition. The aim of the research was to assess the record of holistic precept and practice and to make it more accessible to colleagues in the field of complementary medicine. Extensive quotations from the Hippocratic writers were included in order that the texts could be allowed to speak for themselves as far as possible. The research was conducted under the supervision of a classics scholar and an Ayurvedic medicine scholar. To enhance the investigation, a comparative method was adopted using a classic text of Ayurveda, the *Charaka Samhita*. Ayurveda is a holistic system, both historically contemporary with that of Hippocrates and extant today. Due to restraints of time and space, this chapter will concentrate on the findings in the Greek record. A more extended discussion of the research is to be found elsewhere (Pitman 2004).

THE ORIGINS OF WESTERN HERBAL MEDICINE

The research was prompted by a perceived lack of connection on the part of practitioners in the Western tradition with any historical roots. This contrasts with the situation among Chinese and Ayurvedic practitioners. Furthermore, the many different Western disciplines – osteopathy, homeopathy, herbal medicine, nutrition, naturopathy, massage – can appear as discrete, separate and lacking any common principles or philosophy (Foundation for Integrated Medicine 1997). By and large, the tendency is to regard Eastern forms of traditional medicine as grounded in an encompassing philosophy, and as historically holistic. The general public too is today more familiar with concepts of *yin*, *yang* and *Qi*, or *prana* and *dosas*, than with *pneuma* and humours.

In addition, interest in the corpus was prompted by reading such passages as the following description of how medicine was conceived and practised in ancient Greece:

"Perhaps you ... have heard what good doctors say when a patient comes to them with sore eyes ... They say ... that to think that one could ever treat the head by itself without the whole body is quite foolish. On that principle then, they apply their regimens to the entire body and attempt to treat and heal the part in conjunction with the whole (to holon)."
                              (Plato: Charmides, 156 BCE, cited in Watt 1987)

This fifth-century BCE report on ancient medical practice is striking in its similarity to the approach of modern practitioners of complementary holistic medicine. Is it possible that the origins for the contemporary holistic approach are to be found in 'that principle' on which these ancient Greek physicians based their work? What else is there in their work that is still either germane to, or reflected in, contemporary practice?

The writings of Hippocratic physicians have been studied for many centuries, but not from the point of view of a modern practitioner. The method used was, first, to identify key concepts of contemporary holistic practice, then to 'interrogate the texts' or examine the record as found in the corpus and related texts for evidence of such ideas.

Holistic concepts of today were identified as:

- the vital force
- the wisdom of the body
- the mind–body–spirit connection
- the relationship between health and disease
- treating to support healing processes and balance the body

- treating the individual not the disease
- the participatory role of the patient; the patient–practitioner partnership.

Featherstone & Forsyth (1997, pp. 24-27) outlined the distinctive approach of a holistic as opposed to the biomedical model as follows:

- responding to patients as a whole (body, mind and spirit) within the context of their environment (family, culture, and ecology)
- a willingness to use a wide range of interventions, from drugs and surgery to meditation and diet
- an emphasis on a more participatory relationship between doctor and patient
- awareness of the impact of the 'health' of the practitioner on the patient. ('Physician heal thyself.')

THE HIPPOCRATIC CORPUS

The name Hippocrates is fundamental to Western medicine. Various sayings such as 'you are what you eat' are often attributed to him but seldom, if ever, are references given so that one can look it up and find out what else he might have said. Few today outside the realms of classical scholarship appreciate the scope or detail of ancient medicine. Classical scholarship is, of course, necessary to interpreting the evidence and very welcome; yet it has its limitations.

Most classics scholars are, for instance, embedded in the scientific culture of the modern West, and this is reflected in how they view ancient medical practice. Sometimes the ancient writings are examined by medical doctors, but these tend to concentrate on the ethical aspects and discount the efficacy of the methods. One scholar noted that the nineteenth-century physician and classicist M. P. E. Littré was 'the last commentator for whom Hippocrates was alive and meaningful in day to day medical practice' (Smith 1979, p. 31).

For those not familiar with Hippocrates, as I was not, it is necessary to explain a little about this early source of ancient medicine. Although we know that there was a famous physician of the fifth century BCE called Hippocrates, today it is not certain whether he is the author of any of the writings that are collectively called the Hippocratic corpus. (Scholars have considered this 'Hippocratic question' for several decades without finding a solution.) What *is* known is that the roughly 60 treatises that comprise the corpus were written by several authors in Ionian Greek over a period of about 150 years in the fifth to fourth centuries BCE. They were produced in an era when writing was relatively new and itself undergoing dramatic change, as ideas were beginning to be expressed in prose rather than poetic forms.

Different, sometimes completely contradictory, voices and views are represented, which is not surprising given the timescale. Some treatises are considered to be polemical and rhetorical works defending a particular theory of medicine or persuading a lay audience of the distinctive value of the art and craft (*techne*) of medicine; that is, that medicine is worthy of status and recognition. Others are case notes, recording the progress of diseases in individuals. Some are thought to be lectures or information for the training of student physicians. There is no complete agreement among the various authors on either the causes or treatments of disease. However, underlying all the arguing and diversity of opinion and practice, the treatises do convey a foundation of agreement about disease and wellness (Jones 1972, p. xxix).

A theme found throughout the variety of the treatises, though expressed very individually, is a reverence for the divineness of nature (Temkin 1995). Like Ayurveda, which was closely related to movements in philosophical thought emerging from the *Upanishads*, Greek medicine emerged from that paradigm shift (Kuhn 1970) in thinking that occurred in sixth-century BCE Greek thought. The corpus shows the influence of this 'revolution of wisdom' (Lloyd 1987) by the *phusikoi*, a diverse group of thinkers who 'invented' the idea of the naturalness of nature. It is important to emphasize this point in relation to the corpus because, since the scientific revolution, a cultural bias has tended to play down medicine's philosophical–spiritual side and highlight only the protoscientific aspects. Greek medicine was in fact embedded in a philosophical discipline and way of life that influenced all that the physician did.

THE STUDY OF NATURE

Rather than explaining the universe and physical phenomenon with reference to anthropomorphized deities and supernatural demons, these early Greek innovators sought to understand and explain phenomena through a study of natural forces. Hence the term they used for their activity was *phusikon*, the study of '*phusis*' or nature. Ionian thinkers such as Thales, Anaxagoras, Anaximander and Heraclitus, followed later by others from western Greece (modern southern Italy) such as Pythagoras, Empedocles and Alcmaeon, gave very individual accounts, but, taken together, they represent what has been called the spiritual discovery of the *kosmos*. As a corollary, human life could be viewed as free from magic or supernatural interventions. This philosophical and medical journey was part of man's movement away from a magico-religious view to a rational one. But, importantly, to these ancient thinkers rationalism and reason were concepts that were not set in opposition to divinity or spirituality but part and parcel of the divine nature. The Greek word for universe, *kosmos*, means both order and beauty and it was conceived of as the *sphairos*, great sphere, and the *holon*, or divine whole. The *kosmos* and nature are intelligent, orderly and rational and are intelligible to humans precisely because humans share the faculty and attribute of divine reason. Philosophers such as Pythagoras, Empedocles and Plato also believed that the divine spark in human nature was a particle of the divine, and that through special training and ways of living, men and women could become 'assimilated to the divine'.

Box 7.1 details the Greek cosmic scheme.

Nature, the creative vital force, unfolds out of universal first principles: the *archai* or elements of *Aither*, Air, Fire, Water and Earth. These elements have basic qualities or powers (*dynameis*): heat, cold, wetness and dryness. They

---

Box 7.1   The Greek cosmic scheme

This presentation of the *kosmos* is based on the text *Empedocles, the extant fragments* (Wright 1981). Empedocles' philosophy greatly influenced some medical writers, such as the author of the *Nature of man* (Jones 1979). The *kosmos* is ordered in different parts:

The kosmos

Holon, the Whole/kosmos/kphairos the sphere/aither

These parts are united in harmony and blended by love.
We know that the sphere 'binds all things fast' (Wright 1981). The eternal, divine unity holds all things in harmony. *Phren iere*, holy mind or wisdom, allows the perfection of mingling, with no separation and with the different parts not subject to change.

Nature

Phusis, nature

This represents the created world of forms. All of nature is derived from the mingling of the four elements, or roots, or *archai*. These are Earth, Water, Fire and Air. The elements are blended in different proportions in the different forms of the world (e.g. plants or animals). However, such blending is never perfect, as strife is pulling them apart while a remnant of love holds them together. These ideas are discussed in Plato's *Symposium*.

The human body

The human body includes *daimon*, the god within, and *nous*, understanding. This intelligence, *nous*, dwells in the blood around the heart. The body is formed of elements, by love. The elements mingle to form the body, either male or female, with parts (limbs, bones, hair) and organs (heart, skin, nostrils). The elements enable sense and perception (seeing, smelling and hearing), and also the tastes (sweet, bitter, sharp and hot). Blood represents the most perfect blending of elements within the body.

The authors of the *Nature of man*, describing 'what is' say that the elements mix to form the humours of the body. Some particular part, 'this one', is not one element or another, as other writers have said. Rather, man is formed of many constituents, particularly phlegm, choler, blood and melancholy. These make up the nature of his body and, through these, he feels pain or enjoys health (Jones 1979).

exist in all of nature from the stars and planets to within the human body. Change and disruption are part of nature's order, as the elements undergo *krasis*, mingling, to establish *harmonia*, degrees of separation, then mingle again in the cycle of life. According to Empedocles, and later Plato, harmonious mingling is accomplished through the agency of love. These ideas are found reflected in the medical writings.

GREEK IDEAS OF THE HUMAN BODY

From the concern with the nature of the *kosmos* developed a focus on the 'nature of man'. The corpus reveals that, although there were different lines of thought among physicians, there was general agreement about the fundamentals (Jones 1972). In the human body, the *archai* are manifest as vital breath, vital fire, and vital fluids or humours: *pneuma*, *thermon*, and *chumos*. Thus man is a microcosm of the universal macrocosm.

In scholarship, much has been made of the fact that some medical writers deplored the intrusion of philosophy into medicine, seeing this as an example of a view more like that of modern science. They have been at pains to minimize or regret the connection between philosophy and medicine (Longrigg 1993). Another view is that such authors' statements are less an attempt to separate medicine from philosophy than to emphasize that the physicians had their own traditions of holism, rational study and knowledge about nature distinct from those of any particular philosophical school. The physicians were themselves investigating the *kosmos* as it appeared before them in their patients and in the forces that acted on them. The method they employed was a medical reasoning, *logismos iatrikos*, which was part of a distinct medical tradition (Lain Entralgo 1970). This method, physicians felt, made medicine worthy of the status of a *techne* within Greek society.

The method involved careful observation and above all discerning the truth behind the superficial layer of phenomena. Although received wisdom considers ancient medicine to be unscientific, this method is, I submit, essentially the same as that employed by physicists, a method based on inference. Physicists cannot directly observe the phenomena they study, only their consequences. They envisage models based on their observations, conduct activities based on these models, and get results that are repeatable and predictable. Similarly, the ancient physicians gained information by inference from very careful observation of the signs and activities of the body (supplemented with some knowledge of anatomy and physiology), and conceived a model of explanation and functioning derived from it. They conducted therapies based on this model that in an acceptable number of circumstances were successful, repeatable and predictable. This experience over time gave them the confidence that their method was worthwhile.

Any explanation given had to be faithful to the *logos* (truth, reality) of nature. For physicians, the nature of the human body was the reality to which the logos of the physician should above all be applied. The *Regimen 1* states that it is important to know the 'nature of man in general . . . from what things he is originally composed and discern by what parts he is controlled' (Jones 1979, p. 227). The *Art XI* emphasizes that what escapes the eyesight is mastered by the eye of the mind (Jones 1981, p. 211). Thus medicine involved a philosophical discipline of observation, discernment, and forming a therapeutic strategy combined with the practical skills to carry it out. It was a way of life devoted to the logos:

"transplant wisdom into medicine and medicine into wisdom. For a physician who is a lover of wisdom is the equal of a god. Between wisdom and medicine there is no gulf fixed."

(Jones 1981, p. 287)

THE CONCEPTUALIZATION OF HOLISM

Some examples are given in Box 7.2 of how holistic medicine is conceptualized in the medical writings. The reader needs to bear in mind that any excerpt may illustrate more than one holistic concept since it is difficult to separate the many strands of thought present.

Concepts of health and disease and the physician's role

The physician is seen as acting in concert with nature's healing force to restore wholeness, the shared goal. The body's response to disease is itself a manifestation of nature's intelligent healing power and was well studied by physicians.

Although the physicians recognized, studied and documented many different diseases (e.g. *Diseases and affections*), ultimately disease was attributed to some imbalance in the organism caused from either the external or internal environment. *Breaths* states that:

"of all diseases the fashion is the same but the seat varies, so while diseases are thought to be entirely unlike one another owing to the difference in their seat, in reality all have one essence and cause."

(Jones 1981, pp. 229, 231)

A corollary of this idea was that, as we have seen, the whole person was to be treated, not just the specific disease or symptom. Health was seen as a state of positive well-being that needs care and attention to maintain. It is for this reason that physicians were keen to recommend changes in the patient's daily routine of diet, labour and exercise in order to maintain balance and health and prevent the return of disease.

An impairment of the digestive process, *pepsis* – a concoction or inner cooking – was another way imbalance could be created. By the innate digestive fire, *thermon*, foods are transformed, mingled and mixed together, *krasis*,

Box 7.2 Conceptualization of holism

Examples of vital force, mind–body–soul connections, the wisdom of the body, divine nature and holism in medical writings

Divine nature is manifest in the body primarily as vital *pneuma*. *Breaths* and *The sacred disease* relate that *pneuma* is the source of life, health and, when blocked or imbalanced, the original cause of all disease:

> What can take place without it? In what is it not present? What does it not accompany? ... there is nothing that is empty of air ... for mortals too this is the cause of life and the cause of disease in the sick.
>
> (Jones 1972, p. 83)

Man is composed of cosmic elements, has a soul and is connected to the whole

Regimen 1 declares that:

> ... into man there enters a soul having fire and water ... All things are set in due order both the soul of man and likewise his body ... Soul is the same in all living creatures although the body is different ... All things take place for men through a divine necessity ...
>
> (Jones 1972, pp. 241, 239, 267, 237)

Humours

> The boundary of death is passed when the heat of the soul has risen above the navel to the part above the diaphragm, all the moisture has been burnt up ... there passes away all at once the breath of the heat (wherefrom the whole was constructed) into the whole again, partly through the flesh and partly through the breathing organs in the head, whence we call it the breath of life, and the soul, leaving the tabernacle of the body gives up the cold, mortal image to bile, blood, phlegm and flesh ...
>
> (Jones 1981, p. 81)

The whole and the parts

> Cobblers divide wholes into parts and make the parts wholes; cutting and stitching they make sound what is rotten. Man too has the same experience. Wholes are divided into parts, and from union of the parts wholes are formed. By stitching and cutting, that which is rotten in men is healed by the physician's art: to do away with that which causes pain, and by taking away the cause of his suffering to make him sound. Nature of herself knows how to do these things. . . In other respects too nature is the same as the physician's art.
>
> (Jones 1981, p. 253)

Nature as healing power

The body's nature is the physician in disease. Nature finds the way for herself, not from thought. Well trained, readily and without instruction, nature does what is needed.

(Smith 1994, p. 255)

Nutriment

Nature is sufficient in all, for all.

(Jones 1972, p. 347)

The mind–body connectedness of the human organism

The author of *Breaths* states that when the blood is altered the intelligence changes also (Jones 1981, p. 248). *Epidemics* notices that:

Anger contracts the heart and the lungs and draws the hot and the moist substances into the head. Contentment releases the heart and those substances.

(Smith 1994, p. 257)

In another example, it is observed in the *Humours* that:

States of mind before and after changes . . . Fears, shame, pain, pleasure, passion to each of these the appropriate member of the body responds by its action.

(Jones 1981, p. 81)

Treating the mind and the body

There are several examples of physicians treating patients at the mental level. For example, in *Regimen IV*, the physician recommends the patient to attend the theatre to see a comedy – perhaps the first recorded instance of laughter therapy (Jones 1979, p. 433).

---

so that no one stands alone, *monarchia*, and becomes disproportionately strong. *Krasis* renders foods suitable for absorption and nourishment. For several authors, diet and regimen were the main focus for diagnosis and treatment.

Similarly, the *humours* or vital fluids could cause disease if they became imbalanced through the isolation of one or more of their elements. The humours were the manifestations of cosmic elements and were understood to correspond with times of the day, seasons, climates and the ages of human life. People's lifestyle habits, personality or character disposition, eating habits, and mental and emotional patterns were reflected in their humoral balance. In diagnosing and treating disease, the physician would strive to understand individual patients' *phusis*, or constitution, and unique blend of humours, and to give treatment accordingly.

Erixymachus, the physician attending Plato's *Symposium*, describes medicine as being concerned with the principles of love at work in the body. A skilful doctor is one who can implant love in a body that needs it, enabling the different elements to cease from hostitily and develop mutual affections and love: 'The original nature is the effective thing. One must consider also what comes from way of life' (Smith 1994, p. 27).

For the author of *Regimen 1* it is also important to know that: 'nature of man in general ... from what things he is originally composed and discern by what parts he is controlled' (Jones 1981, p. 227). For this author, man was primarily composed of fire and water:

"Fire has the hot and the dry, water the cold and the moist. Mutually, too, fire has the moist from water, for in fires there is moisture and water has the dry from fire, for there is dryness in water also."

(Jones 1979, p. 233)

For the author of *Nature of man*, whose medical model was one of four humours, the method of medicine involves constitutional diagnosis and treatment:

"The physician must set himself against the established character of the disease, of constitutions, of seasons and of ages... One should carry out treatment only after examination of the patient's constitution, age, physique, season of the year and the fashion of the disease, sometimes taking away, sometimes adding and so making changes in drugging or in regimen to suit the several conditions of age, season, physique, and disease."

(Jones 1981, p. 25)

By working in this way, the physician was following nature: 'Nature of herself knows how to do these things ... In other respects too nature is the same as the physician's art' (Jones 1981, p. 253).

THE PATIENT'S ROLE

The patient must be involved in the healing process, since, as part of nature, patients are being influenced by their surroundings. In order to keep well, they must take responsibility for adopting a beneficial *diaita*, diet, and *bios*, mode of living. Even mental habits were recognized as being important to health. Health was enhanced by following the order and regularity of the cycles of nature. Since the body was believed to have an intelligent self-healing mechanism, the patient's role was to support this healing force of nature so far as possible:

"The patient himself must bring about a cure by combating the cause of the disease, for in this way will be removed that which caused the disease in the body... If [patients] understood their diseases, they would never have fallen into them."

(Jones 1979, p. 37; 1981, p. 211)

The physician's duty was to involve patients in the process of healing and help them learn how to keep well:

"Now to learn by themselves how their own sufferings come about and cease, and the reasons why they get worse or better is not an easy task for ordinary folk, but if you fail to put your hearers in this condition you will miss reality (ontas)."

(Jones 1972, pp. 15, 17)

Food and diet

Food and dietary regimen are the subject of many of the treatises, as both cause and cure for disease. Each food or drink had a certain power or quality based on its taste and nature, and this knowledge was used to balance the body through regimen and treatment principles of 'like to like', and 'opposites to balance opposites'. Treatment was focused on ensuring the functioning of the organs of elimination in order that toxins (*perissomata*) produced from wrong regimen might be removed. *Plethoras* (excesses) were eliminated by therapies such as fasting or therapeutic foods, purging the digestive tract with laxative drugs, cleansing the body with enemas, sweating, or diuretics and prescriptions of exercise. Depletions (deficiencies) were restored with diet, massage, rest and gentle exercise. With such therapies, physicians imitated nature and helped the patient's body to do what nature intended, but in a controlled way.

As a specific example, the research on which this chapter is based looked at ways in which Hippocratic and Ayurvedic physicians conceived and treated fevers. Such diseases feature prominently in texts in both traditions, and similar treatment strategies are used: rest and a light, fluid diet of barley *ptsane*, a gruel (Greece) or rice *kitcharee* (India). Today such medicinal foods are still considered to be cleansing, antipyretic and nutritive. Some 300 herbs are mentioned in the corpus and the physician was expected to know:

"the characteristics of drugs, from what one comes what kinds of things. For they are not all equally good, but different characteristics are good in different circumstances."

(Smith 1994, p. 51)

THE PROBLEMATIC CONCEPT OF 'HUMOURS'

The treatises of the corpus do not reflect agreement among physicians about the number and importance of the humours. In some, a bipolar model of *bile* and *phlegm* is used. In others, *water* is given as a third humour. Several treatises, most prominently *Nature of man* (Jones 1979), find that the human is composed of four humours: *bile, phlegm, blood* and *melancholy*. Three of these are readily seen to be bodily fluids but the inclusion of melancholy or, literally, dark bile has long puzzled medical historians because it is not an obvious bodily fluid. From my examination of the treatises, I have concluded that the somewhat later inclusion of melancholy as a humour represented a development and a refinement in Greek medical thought, under the influence of Empedocles, to accommodate physicians' increasing knowledge and experience (Jones 1981). Experience had grown particularly with relation to consciousness, environmental factors and diseases that involved irregularity of the natural order. In *Nature of man* (Jones 1981) the qualities of melancholy, coolness and dryness are associated with those of the season autumn, and with periods of change in general. In a variety of treatises, diseases reported as melancholic are consistent with some derangement of the mind, conditions of nervous pathology, late stages of fevers or chronic ulcers – conditions when the body's vital heat, air or fluids have been dried, pathologically changed or threatened by melancholy's dryness or coldness.

Melancholy was a word and concept long extant in popular Greek culture for madness and derangements of the natural order. Likewise, consciousness had been associated with the *pneuma* as present in the blood humour. Coldness and dryness were part of the intelligent order of nature, but if present to excess in the body became threatening to the vital air, moisture and warmth, and thus caused disease. So, the four-humour model represented a means of including in medical reasoning a more developed idea of the functions of vital air, perceiving in the warm, moist blood humour the qualities of vital air in its optimal state and in the melancholy humour the cooling and drying qualities of air. In doing so, the model makes explicit the physicians' knowledge of the mind–body–spirit reality of human nature. It reflects the greater detail of understanding of the processes of change in the body that physicians had gained through experience. It is a model that is more dynamic and comprehensive than previous bipolar or tripolar models, since it takes into account finer nuances of seasons, climates, ageing and mental–spiritual health.

The importance placed by the Hippocratic physicians on the health of humours, the vital fluids that embody the mental, emotional and spiritual aspects of the human being, shows that they were keenly aware of what today has been termed psychoneuroimmunology. Humoralism has long been dismissed by medical science as outdated but, in the light of this study, takes on a renewed relevance. In their own terms, the ancient physicians understood that immunity is dependent on humoral – that is, fluid-borne and fluid-mediated – mechanisms (see Brooks et al 1962, Nutton 1993). Keeping the humours – the blood, bile, lubricating fluids and hormonal secretions – healthy and in balance was, and is still, the key to health and long life.

CONCLUSION

The Hippocratic corpus is well worth studying for insights into the maintenance of health, the process of disease and the practice of the healer that are still relevant to the complementary medicine practitioner. It is hoped that other practitioners will discover more by reading these treatises. Key ideas of the contemporary holistic approach are found powerfully expressed in the ancient medical system of Western culture. A comparison of ideas of holism in the Hippocratic corpus and Ayurveda strengthens the appreciation that the theory and practice of Greek medicine were grounded in an equally comprehensive spiritual–philosophical base. Finally, the fact that such concepts are found in the corpus provides a point of unification for otherwise apparently diverse and disconnected disciplines that goes beyond herbal medicine. Such disciplines with their origins in Greek thinking include homeopathy and massage as well as herbal medicine. This study shows that we are in fact inheritors of a common, and deep, source of holism.

References

Brooks C M, Gilbert, J L, Levey, H A 1962 Humours, hormones and neurosecretions. State University of New York, New York

Featherstone C, Forsyth L 1997 Medical marriage: the new partnership, Findhorn Press, London

Foundation for Integrated Medicine 1997 Integrated health care: a discussion document. Foundation for Integrated Medicine, London

Jones W H S 1972 Hippocrates, vol 1. Loeb classical library. Harvard University Press and Heinemann, Cambridge

Jones W H S 1979 Hippocrates, vol 4. Loeb classical library. Harvard University Press and Heinemann, Cambridge

Jones W H S 1981 Hippocrates, vol 2. Loeb classical library. Harvard University Press and Heinemann, Cambridge

Kuhn T S 1970 The structure of scientific revolutions. University of Chicago Press, Chicago

Lain Entralgo P 1970 The therapy of the word in classical antiquity. Yale University Press, New Haven

Lloyd G E R 1987 Revolutions of wisdom: studies in the claims and practice of ancient Greek science. University of California Press, Berkeley

Longrigg J 1993 Greek rational medicine. Routledge, London

Nutton V 1993 Humoralism. In: Bynum W F, Porter R (eds) Companion encyclopedia of the history of medicine. Routledge, London

Pitman V 2004 Sources of holism in Ancient Greek and Indian medicine. Motilal Barnasidas, Delhi

Smith W D 1979 The Hippocratic tradition. Cornell University Press, Ithaca

Smith W D 1994 Hippocrates, vol 7. Loeb classical library. Harvard University Press and Heinemann, Cambridge

Temkin O 1995 Hippocrates in a world of pagans and Christians. Johns Hopkins University Press, Baltimore

Watt D 1987 The Charmides Plato. In: Saunders T J (ed) Early Socratic dialogues, vol MX. Penguin, Harmondsworth

Wright MR 1981 Empedocles, the extant fragments. Yale University Press, Cambridge

Further reading

Potter P 1995 Hippocrates, vol 8. Loeb classical library. Harvard University Press and Heinemann, Cambridge

Sharma R K, Dash B 1985 The Caraka-Samhita. Chowkhamba Orientalia, Varanasi

Problems with knowledge, education and culture in the development of the herbal medicine profession

8

Patient safety and practitioner identity:
the move towards statutory self-regulation

R Michael Pittilo

OVERVIEW

The Herbal Medicine Regulatory Working Group (HMRWG) was established by the Department of Health (DH), the Prince of Wales's Foundation for Integrated Health (PoWFIH) and the European Herbal Practitioners Association (EHPA) in January 2002. It was formed as a direct consequence of the recommendations within the House of Lords' Select Committee on Science and Technology's report on complementary and alternative medicine (2000) and the Government response (Department of Health 2001a) to it. For many practitioners, the report from the House of Lord's Select Committee (2000) was welcomed and viewed as the next step towards the statutory regulation of the profession. It was the culmination of over a decade of activity directed towards statutory regulation. A significant number of practitioners, however, questioned the need for statutory self-regulation, arguing that voluntary regulation provided sufficient safeguards for the public. Events described in this chapter should be viewed in this context.

INTRODUCTION

History will confirm the House of Lords' Select Committee's report (2000) as an important and significant milestone in the statutory regulation of herbal medicine. It defined herbal medicine, or phytotherapy as it is sometimes called, as 'a system of medicine which uses various remedies derived from plants and plant extracts to treat disorders and maintain good health'. The report, and perhaps this may be seen as the least helpful aspect of an otherwise valuable contribution, classified complementary and alternative medicine (CAM) therapies into three groups. Therapies assigned to Group 1 were considered to be the principal disciplines, each with an individual diagnostic approach and incorporating the most organized professions. These therapies were also considered those most likely to respond to research on effectiveness, with NHS provision for these therapies increasing. The report assigned to Group 2 those therapies that are used as complementary to conventional orthodox medical treatments. Although some of them can be accessed via the NHS, the report concluded that more work needs to be undertaken to develop their regulatory structures and to research their specific effects. Within this group, and therapies assigned to Group 3, the report concluded that there was considerable diversity of standards, with unacceptable fragmentation in some therapies. The therapies assigned to Group 3 were defined as those purporting to offer diagnostic information and treatment, but mainly favouring a philosophical approach with indifference to the scientific principles of conventional medicine. Group 3 therapies were further separated into Group 3a, long-established and traditional systems of healthcare, and Group 3b, covering other CAM disciplines. The most critical statement within the report of the Group 3 therapies was that for many of them no evidence base exists and that they should not be supported until convincing evidence of efficacy is obtained through well-designed trials.

The report from the House of Lords (2000) assigned herbal medicine to Group 1 along with acupuncture, chiropractic, homoeopathy and osteopathy. As osteopathy and chiropractic were already statutorily regulated, the inclusion of herbal medicine in this group conferred status upon the profession that was broadly welcomed. The report recognized the popularity of CAM amongst the public and supported the statutory regulation of herbal medicine, which was identified as posing particular challenges for public health. Within the United Kingdom, it is estimated that about 30% of the population has used herbal medicines (Thomas et al 2001). The report also supported the statutory regulation of acupuncture and considered that, in time, regulation might also be appropriate for homeopathy. The report recognized that there was considerable diversity of standards amongst the professions within CAM and that, for some therapies, the public was at risk from practitioners with inadequate or inappropriate training. Within the herbal medicine profession there were already well-developed regulatory structures, unlike many other CAM therapies that remain disorganized with no consensus about regulation.

In recommending that herbal medicine should be statutorily regulated, the House of Lords' report (2000) concluded that it met their key criteria. These included risk to the public through poor practice, a voluntary regulation system and a credible evidence base. With respect to the latter, the report does acknowledge that the evidence for the efficacy of herbal medicine is patchy. However, as far as protecting the public from practitioners using herbal medicine and acupuncture was concerned, the House of Lords' report (2000) did pose some difficulties. The inclusion of CAM therapies using herbal products as medicines, as well as those practising acupuncture, in Groups 2 and 3 meant that they were not candidates for statutory regulation. Maharishi Ayurvedic medicine and Ayurvedic medicine were assigned to Group 2 and Chinese herbal medicine and Traditional Chinese Medicine (TCM) were assigned to Group 3. In determining that, for these therapies, criteria for statutory regulation had not been met, only partial protection would be afforded to the public from practitioners using herbal products as medicines. A similar issue existed for acupuncture, as there were therapies separate from acupuncture in Group 1 that use this modality, with consequential issues for patient protection. To illustrate this, practitioners of TCM (Group 3) use both herbal medicine and acupuncture.

The Government response to the House of Lords' Select Committee report on CAM (Department of Health 2001a) supported the recommendation proposing the statutory regulation of herbal medicine and acupuncture, and considered that this should be undertaken as soon as practicable. It went as far as stating that it would be prepared to consider the possibility of extending statutory regulation to other therapies if there was a case for it. Establishing the case would include the existence of a unified professional body, with the support of most members of the profession for pursuing that option. The response acknowledged, for example, that members of the aromatherapy profession had expressed an interest in becoming statutorily regulated.

The Government response (Department of Health 2001a) resolved the difficulty over regulation resulting from the grouping in the House of Lords' report by determining that there was scope, in certain circumstances, for therapies to be allied for a specific purpose across the boundaries of the proposed groupings. It determined that, for the purposes of professional self-regulation, aspects of the therapies listed in Group 3 that use herbal remedies could come together within a federal grouping of therapies in Group 1. These could be considered under the general heading of herbal medicine whilst still retaining their individual identities and traditions. The emphasis on retention of identity was to be very important in determining the workings of the HMRWG. The Government response (Department of Health 2001a) determined that herbal medicine and acupuncture should, in the interests of patients, both work as quickly as possible towards statutory regulation under the Health Act 1999. Critically, the Government response allowed for the inclusion of therapies using herbal products as medicines apart from those assigned to Group 1 in the House of Lords' report nevertheless to be involved in the process leading towards statutory self-regulation.

Lastly, the House of Lords' report expressed concern about the safety implications of an unregulated herbal sector and urged that all legislative avenues be explored to ensure better control of this unregulated sector in the interests of the public health. The Government response acknowledged that, for products classified as medicines, there was a weakness in the regulatory arrangements for unlicensed herbal remedies provided for under Section 12(2) of the Medicines Act 1968. Herbal remedies are covered elsewhere in this book (Chapter 9) and will not be discussed here, except to note that the terms of reference of the HMRWG were adapted in order to address this issue. A key aspect of the Government response was to facilitate discussion amongst herbal interest groups to consider the way forward. The HMRWG made recommendations on the regulation of herbal remedies made up to meet individual needs and supplied to the public after a personal consultation under the provisions of Section 12(1) of the Medicines Act 1968.

TERMS OF REFERENCE

The HMRWG's terms of reference were therefore informed by both the House of Lords' report on CAM (2000) and the Government response (2001a). They were framed by the DH with the PoWFIH and the EHPA and encapsulated in a scoping paper owned by the DH. The response of the DH to the House of Lords' report and the Government response was to establish a regulatory working group for herbal medicine (HMRWG) and a parallel working group for acupuncture (ARWG). The terms of reference were drafted by the stakeholders and revised with their agreement by the HMRWG (Box 8.1). The significant change was the introduction of the second important requirement for us to make recommendations for ensuring the safety and quality of herbal remedies supplied under Section 12(1).

Box 8.1 The Herbal Medicine Regulatory Working Group

The confirmed terms of reference for the HMRWG were to:

1. produce a report that examines the options for achieving the successful statutory regulation of the herbal medicine profession as a whole, and makes recommendations that will form the basis for a wider consultation by the government and subsequently for the legislation that will enable the statutory regulation of the herbal medicine profession
2. in the light of the recommendations for the statutory regulation of the profession and the current Medicines and Healthcare Products Regulatory Agency (formerly the Medicines Control Agency) review of Section 12(1) of the Medicines Act 1968, make recommendations for ensuring the safety and quality of herbal remedies supplied under Section 12(1).

The key objectives for the HMRWG were to:

1. support and promote moves towards unification within a federal structure of the herbal practitioner profession
2. produce a report, as outlined above in the terms of reference, by April 2003
3. recommend within the report whether any changes to medicines law relating to the supply of unlicensed herbal remedies following one-to-one consultation may be desirable in order to assure the consumer as to the safety and quality of these medicines.

MEMBERSHIP

I was interviewed for the position of lay Chair of the HMRWG in late 2001 and appointed by the DH to this position. The HMRWG formally commenced its work in January 2002.

Membership of the HMRWG had been determined by the principal stakeholders (that is the DH, the PoWFIH and the EHPA) and was not in any sense influenced by the newly appointed Chair.

The following organizations were represented on the HMRWG:

- College of Practitioners of Phytotherapy (CPP)
- Association of Master Herbalists (AMH)

- National Institute of Medical Herbalists (NIMH)
- European Herbal Practitioners Association (EHPA)
- British Society of Chinese Medicine (BSCM)
- Register of Chinese Herbal Medicine (RCHM)
- International Register of Consultant Herbalists (IRCH)
- Unified Register of Herbal Practitioners (URHP)
- Ayurvedic Medical Association (AMA)
- Association of Traditional Chinese Medicine (ATCM)
- British Association of Accredited Ayurvedic Practitioners (BAAAP) and British Ayurvedic Medical Council (BAMC).

The Royal Pharmaceutical Society of Great Britain (RPSGB) was represented on the working group, as was the chair of the Education Committee of the EHPA. There was representation from each of the stakeholder organizations (that is the DH, the PoWFIH and the EHPA). The HMRWG had, in addition to the lay Chair, three lay members. The representative from the Royal Pharmaceutical Society also played a role as a lay member as far as herbal medicine was concerned. Lastly, the Chair was supported by a Vice-Chair, who was a member of the National Institute of Medical Herbalists (NIMH), and a Project Director of the EHPA. The Chair of the HMRWG was accountable to the stakeholder organizations. Both the Chair and the lay members were provided with an induction into herbal medicine prior to commencement of the HMRWG.

It is clear that the stakeholders determined that the representation should be wide and inclusive. Although the membership was large, it did mean that almost all elements of the herbal medicine profession were represented on the HMRWG.

Box 8.2 details the roles of the different stakeholders.

Box 8.2   The role of the stakeholders

Department of Health

The DH played a key role in supporting the HMRWG. It took the lead in establishing the group, preparing a scoping document to initiate and guide the working group and, not least, provided a framework within which the working group could operate. The DH resourced the working group by providing honoraria for lay members, with the exception of the Chair, and covering travelling expenses. The DH also provided accommodation for the working group for one residential meeting towards the end of our deliberations. The DH provided extensive advice but did not influence the process. The working group was encouraged to develop its own recommendations, taking account of what would be best for herbal medicine.

The Prince of Wales's Foundation for Integrated Health

The PoWFIH played a major role in facilitating the deliberations of both the Herbal Medicine Regulatory Working Group and the Acupuncture Regulatory

---

Box 8.2   (Continued)

Working Group. It provided a representative to both groups, organized through its regulatory programme some helpful conferences and seminars, both during the life of the working group and following its reporting, and provided guidance to the Chair and support for the lay members. The PoWFIH provided an honorarium for the Chair during the first year of the working group, which was not taken personally but paid direct to his host institution, in compensation for time out of work. The PoWFIH had a pivotal role to play in supporting the publication of the HMRWG report, including financially supporting the production of the document, including the costs of copyediting and publication. Without the involvement of the PoWFIH, public and practitioner awareness of the consultation would have been much less widespread.

European Herbal Practitioners Association

The EHPA, again, played a key role including financially supporting the deliberations of the working group. It is a large and effective federal organization that has worked hard for close to a decade, building consensus around the regulation of herbal medicine. It brought to the HMRWG a draft core curriculum, proposals for continuing professional development, accreditation guidelines and a code of ethics. These were all debated and modified during the life of the working group. The Chair of the EHPA was an invaluable source of guidance and expertise and had responsibility for chairing the Herbal Medicine Subcommittee of the working group. The DH was determined that the views of the herbal medicine profession should be considered by the HMRWG and influence our recommendations. The EHPA had a pivotal role in brokering consensus across the organizations representing herbal medicine, although it was much more difficult with the non-affiliated bodies. Although suspicions of the intentions of the EHPA were always evident, perhaps only I as Chair was aware of how hard this organization worked, both before and during this period, to help enable a consensus.

Medicines and Healthcare Products Regulatory Agency (MHRA) (formerly the Medicines Control Agency)

Although not a stakeholder, the MHRA played a significant role in supporting the HMRWG in framing recommendations on the Reform of Section 12(1) of the Medicines Act 1968.

The EHPA is a federal organization, representing a wide range of organizations from the different herbal medicine traditions. One difficulty from the outset was that two of the organizations on the HMRWG were not affiliated to the EHPA. These were the Association of Traditional Chinese Medicine (ATCM), and the British Association of Accredited Ayurvedic Practitioners (BAAAP) with the associated BAMC. These organizations had, not surprisingly, concerns about the dominance of the influence of the EHPA-affiliated bodies on the HMRWG.

This meant that the working group had to consider, from the start, the question of the legitimacy of the various groups who purported to speak on behalf of the practitioner community. Furthermore, it rendered problematic the notion that the profession could be viewed as a community.

METHOD OF WORKING

The HMRWG met approximately every 2 months from its inception in January 2002 until publication of its reports in September 2003. From the outset, I, as Chair, determined a number of principles that would guide our working to produce the report. Firstly, the Chair was anxious to achieve consensus among the organizations represented on the HMRWG. I determined to do everything possible to ensure that the two organizations that were not affiliated to the EHPA did not feel disadvantaged. Although this was only partially achieved, the lay members had a key role to play within the deliberations of the HMRWG to ensure that the views and concerns of all organizations were heard and not dominated by the majority view within the EHPA. The lay members went to great lengths to work with the non-affiliated organizations, meeting on a number of occasions with representatives who did not share the EHPA view. Some indication of their commitment to doing this was provided by a very significant concern, several months into the deliberations, by members of the EHPA-affiliated organizations that progress within the HMRWG was being frustrated by too much attention being paid to minority viewpoints.

The second principle was the importance of members of the HMRWG consulting with the organizations that they represented. From the outset, it was recognized that the reports from the HMRWG would carry significantly greater influence if they had been widely discussed within the organizations represented on the working group and were broadly supported by the respective memberships. During the operation of the HMRWG, I received a number of communications from organizations that were represented on the working group. The decision was taken, with the agreement of the HMRWG members, that all correspondence from members would be referred to the appropriate representative on the working group. To support members of the HMRWG, the Chair and the Secretary, and on occasions the lay members, attended a range of conferences at the request of the various organizations represented on the working group. This was very valuable, allowing for discussion with a wide range of practitioners and enabling me to engage with the debates and concerns that existed within the represented organizations. It gave myself and lay members a much greater feel for the issues that concerned practitioners in connection with the regulation of herbal medicine, as well as providing an opportunity for practitioners to seek clarity about the deliberations within the working group.

A third principle was that the HMRWG should not work in isolation from an understanding of current health policy. The HMRWG was established at a time of significant policy change affecting the regulation of existing health professionals, along with changing expectations of the different ways of working by orthodox healthcare professionals to deliver effective healthcare. This was an important principle in shaping our recommendations. If we had not taken account of current health policy, and focused solely on the regulation of herbal medicine in isolation, our recommendations might have been very different. The focus of the working group was always brought back to the centrality of the patient, rather than to the interests of different practitioner groupings.

The final principle was that the discussions within the HMRWG should, as far as possible, not be confidential, and that the process for preparing the reports should be transparent. The confirmed minutes of meetings of the HMRWG were made publicly accessible via the DH website.

THE POLICY CONTEXT

Key to the HMRWG was an awareness of current and emerging health policy, particularly in relation to promoting multiprofessional team working and to regulatory reform. The HMRWG was conscious that the orthodox healthcare professions were being challenged as, perhaps, never before. Policy statements implied that professional self-interest had dominated over the needs of patients and challenged the existing approach to workforce planning, encouraging the development of training and education arrangements that were genuinely multiprofessonal (Department of Health 2000a). The policy imperatives all seemed to be encouraging healthcare professionals to look widely at the needs of patients, and at how they interfaced in their practice with other health professionals. From the outset, this influenced thinking on the option of a stand-alone Herbal Council rather than an interprofessional CAM Council.

Pittilo & Ross (1998) did, however, refer to the unstoppable enthusiasm and momentum for education that promotes multiprofessional practice in the UK. They expressed concern about the paucity of the evidence base to demonstrate that shared teaching and learning, at pre- and postregistration levels, results in effective team working upon qualification. They argued that longitudinal studies and further work are necessary to provide sound evidence for curricula designed to lead to multiprofessional working with demonstrable positive effects on patient outcomes. Nevertheless the policy pressure for interprofessional education and training remains strong. Barr (2002) and Freeth et al (2002) have, respectively, reviewed interprofessional education in a health and social care context, and critically reviewed evaluations within the published literature. Difficulties in designing research to demonstrate the effectiveness of interprofessional education to promote improved team working and care are highlighted (Freeth et al 2002).

The NHS plan (Department of Health 2000b) significantly influenced the deliberations of the working group. It stated that there would be reforms to health curricula to give everyone working in the NHS the skills and knowledge to respond effectively to the individual needs of patients. The NHS plan referred to a new core curriculum for all education programmes for NHS staff, joint training across the professions in communication skills and in NHS organizations and principles and, finally, a common foundation programme (Department of Health 2000b). Although it was recognized by the HMRWG that most practitioners of herbal medicine work outside the NHS, it accepted that much of the policy was relevant to all healthcare professionals, regardless of the sources of funding. In particular, the HMRWG felt that for some areas, such as communication skills, the CAM sector had much to contribute to the education and training of orthodox healthcare professionals.

Responding to the NHS plan (Department of Health 2000b) and the consultation document on the future healthcare workforce (Department of Health 2000a), Finch (2000) proposed four possible reasons for the NHS prioritizing interprofessional education and training. These were:

- to enable students to *'know about'* the roles of other professional groups
- to be able to *'work with'* other professionals in teams
- to be able to *'substitute for'* roles traditionally played by other professionals
- to provide flexibility in career routes – *'moving across'*.

All of these have relevance to herbal medicine and the wider CAM professions. Finch argued for clarity of definition, and the need for the NHS to be specific about the desired objectives, and suggested that effective interprofessional education in a health setting might best take place in clinical settings (Finch 2000).

The HMRWG was also aware of the high priority that had been placed upon introducing interprofessional education and training (Pittilo & Ross 1998) to promote and facilitate developments in the multiprofessional team delivery of healthcare. The determination of the DH to influence curricula for preregistration orthodox healthcare professionals was clear. Following publication of the nursing strategy (Department of Health 1999a), NHS Education and Training Consortia (England only) were invited to bid for pilot site status to introduce a new model of nurse education based on the recommendations in the nurse education strategy (Department of Health 1999b), along with those in the United Kingdom Central Council for Nursing, Midwifery and Health Visiting (UKCC) Commission on Nursing and Midwifery Education (1999). Facilitating interprofessional learning and practice was a key requirement for successful bids (Department of Health 1999b).

Although the nursing strategy was the first to be published, more recent strategies have continued to place heavy emphasis on the need for interprofessional training and working. For example, the strategy for the professions in healthcare sciences (Department of Health 2001b) stressed the need for more interprofessional education and training and the creation of a workforce that was flexible, multidisciplinary and competent, as well as being able to practise across traditional professional boundaries. Similarly, the earlier strategy for the allied health professions placed a strong emphasis on interprofessional education and training (Department of Health 2000c). It stated that the allied health professions were at the forefront of interprofessional education and that learning together can give practitioners an understanding of the roles of other professionals, along with team-building skills, at an early stage in the curriculum (Department of Health 2000c). Although the emphasis on the above policy documents has been on the education and training of orthodox healthcare professionals, the purpose of promoting interprofessional working was one with which CAM practitioners could resonate. It was, after all, a feature of CAM possibly more developed than with orthodox health care professionals. The emphasis on improving communication skills, for example, was broadly endorsed. Nevertheless, within the discussions on the HMRWG, the more problematic aspects of interprofessional working were acknowledged, including the relative imbalances of power between the practitioner community and the larger orthodox sector.

The HMRWG was also cognisant of the changes that were taking place with the regulation of other healthcare professions, reflecting government concerns that statutory regulation needed to be modernized and was insufficiently developed to protect the public. Policy has identified the need for regulatory bodies to work together to develop common systems across the professions and to agree standards that put the interests of patients demonstrably at the heart of professional regulation (Department of Health 2001c). The government has determined that professional regulatory bodies must be open, and make improvements based on feedback from patients, their representatives and the public. They must deal with complaints quickly, thoroughly, objectively and in a way that is responsive to the complainant whilst treating fairly the health professional complained against (Department of Health 2001c). These sentiments influenced the deliberations of the HMRWG.

The culmination of these concerns has been the establishment of the Council for the Regulation of Healthcare Professionals (CRHP), which was created partly in response to the Bristol Inquiry (Bristol Royal Infirmary Inquiry 2001). The inquiry identified weaknesses in the current arrangements for professional regulation and supported the concept of an overarching body for the regulation of health professionals.

The timing of the HMRWG was such that it coincided with the creation of new regulatory bodies. The Health Professions Council (HPC) had just been established in 2001, to replace the Council for Professions Supplementary to Medicine. The Nursing and Midwifery Council was established the following year, as the HMRWG was formed, to replace the UKCC. Prior to this, following the Osteopaths Act 1993 and the Chiropractors Act 1994, the General Osteopathic Council and the General Chiropractic Council were established in 1996 and 1998 respectively.

It cannot be overemphasized how an awareness of the debate on the modernization of regulation influenced the deliberations of the HMRWG. The consultation document on establishing the CRHP (Department of Health 2001c) proposed a framework that explicitly put patients' interests first; is open and transparent and allows for robust public scrutiny; is responsive to change; provides for greater integration and coordination between the regulatory bodies and the sharing of good practice and information; and requires the regulatory bodies to conform to principles of good regulation. Although not uncritical of the implications of such a policy agenda, the members of the working group could clearly identify the directions of travel. From the outset, the HMRWG concluded that separate councils for herbal medicine and acupuncture could run counter to the interests of patients, not least by frustrating the delivery of interprofessional care. Furthermore, and of importance in this particular context, practitioners using both acupuncture and herbal products as medicines, as is the case with TCM, would face particular difficulties with separate regulatory bodies.

SAFETY VERSUS EFFICACY

The HMRWG was solely concerned with safety and not with efficacy. The evidence base for herbal medicine is limited (Lewith et al 2003), but there is a commitment across the sector to undertake rigorous research. It has been argued that a strong evidence base should be a requirement for statutory regulation (Ernst 2003). The view of HMRWG was that herbal medicine is at a stage now where the protection of the public will best be served by statutory regulation being introduced in parallel with research directed to improve the evidence base. While not directly relevant to the recommendations of the working group, we did discuss some of the more problematic aspects of research design in relation to the clinical practice of herbal medicine (Chapter 10).

DELIBERATIONS OF THE HERBAL MEDICINE REGULATORY WORKING GROUP

HMRWG was given a clear mandate to recognize and safeguard the individual traditions that make up herbal medicine. Within the working group, the following traditions were represented – Western herbal medicine, Ayurvedic medicine, TCM and Chinese herbal medicine. The HMRWG also considered Tibetan medicine and Maharishi Ayurvedic medicine, but these were not represented on the group. One immediate difficulty arose with TCM, whereby practitioners use both herbal products as medicines and also acupuncture. It was clear from the outset that TCM practitioners were very concerned about their practice being regulated by a Herbal Council, whilst there was discussion taking place separately about regulation for acupuncture.

With regard to the recommendations for ensuring the safety and quality of herbal remedies supplied under Section 12(1) of the Medicines Act (1968), this was handled by creating a Herbal Medicines Subcommittee. The deliberations of this group are outside the remit of this chapter, other than to note that it was expertly chaired and effective in discharging its business.

In framing its recommendations, the HMRWG did consider a range of options. One of these was whether herbal medicine could be included on the HPC. This was rejected for a number of reasons. Herbal medicine was not well established in mainstream healthcare and its identity could be lost within the HPC. A high priority of the working group was to protect the identity of the individual herbal medicine traditions and, again, it was difficult to see how this could be achieved within the HPC. The HMRWG recognized that the HPC was a new organization, with a heavy developmental agenda, and that the criteria for membership might not be met. Lastly, there were several professions already waiting in line to be considered for inclusion within the HPC and the government had indicated that there was some urgency to regulate herbal medicine. However, some contributors to the debate were keen to stress the value of including herbalists within a newly established statutory body.

Similarly, the HMRWG considered the option of separate councils for each distinctive tradition of herbal medicine. This would have been a preferred option for TCM, but was rejected because of the very small number of practitioners, making this an unviable option. The costs would have been prohibitive and it would have been difficult to see how even smaller traditions such as Tibetan medicine could have been accommodated.

This left two possibilities and one of these became the preferred option. The first option was for the establishment of a Herbal Council. This had advantages in that it had been what the herbal profession had aspired to for almost a decade, and it would allow greater identity building. The clear disadvantages were that it would work against interdisciplinary practice and the costs were likely to be prohibitive. The second option was for a CAM Council, with an initial sharing of regulation between herbal medicine and acupuncture. The HMRWG proposed that this could range from simply sharing a building, reducing overhead costs for both professions, through to a close articulation analogous to the way the HPC works. The HMRWG increasingly became less convinced of the benefits of a stand-alone council, favouring instead the idea of a shared CAM Council. Perhaps controversially, it suggested that osteopathy and chiropractic, as well as homeopathy, which there were no current plans to regulate, might consider the benefits of such an arrangement. There was great hesitation within the working group about making this recommendation as we recognized the significant work that had been undertaken by the osteopaths and chiropractors to achieve statutory regulation. However, looking more widely, the representation of these organizations on the new CRHP seemed disproportionate in relation to their size when compared with nursing, medicine or the allied health professions. Lastly, it was felt that the CAM Council could exert greater influence and that costs would be significantly reduced. It took many meetings to reach a consensus on the best way forward, in order to frame the recommendations in our report. The greatest bar to any wider council was the concern that the influence of herbalists might be reduced, or the process to statutory self-regulation be slowed down by including others.

The recommendations from the HMRWG took account of best regulatory practice as has been referred to above and as described within the various government policy documents. The report recognized the importance of having a register of practitioners competent to prescribe and use herbal products, and other materials, as medicines. In view of the requirements of TCM, herbal medicines were extended to include materials of mineral or animal origin. This was not universally supported, particularly by Western herbal practitioners, some of whom have strong personal beliefs about animal rights. The proposed CAM Council would have responsibility for determining minimum levels of education and training, accreditation of educational establishments, continuing professional development, and conduct and disciplinary procedures.

When I met with practitioners, one of the key concerns that was always raised was the costs of regulation. The HMRWG undertook a financial analysis and became convinced that a shared council would greatly reduce the costs to practitioners. In view of CAM being predominantly practised within the private sector, it was likely that the costs to practitioners would have to be transferred to patients. The HMRWG was persuaded by evidence from the existing health regulatory bodies that increasing the size of the council could lead to efficiency savings. This was therefore a strong influence on the formation of our recommendations.

DIFFICULTIES

There were two significant difficulties that were not resolved. The first of these was with Ayurveda. It was clear from the outset that the organizations representing Ayurveda on the HMRWG had very different views between themselves about education and training standards for this tradition. Despite taking advice from the countries of origin of this important tradition (Chapter 9), along with guidance from organizations not represented on the working group including practitioners of Maharishi Ayurvedic Medicine, consensus was not achieved and this was reflected in the final report. This will continue to be a problem unless agreement can be achieved amongst the different organizations representing Ayurveda.

A further difficulty resulted from the HMRWG making recommendations that had implications for acupuncture, when its remit was for herbal medicine. Taking account of the fact that TCM practitioners use acupuncture within their practice, this difficulty was perhaps inevitable. The problem was exacerbated by the HMRWG proposing a shared council with obvious implications for acupuncture, and other CAM professions. Perhaps, with hindsight, it would have been preferable to have established a joint working group or, at least, a formal requirement for the two groups to interface formally. Although the Chairs of the working groups did regularly meet, as did the respective Secretaries, the DH was presented with different reports with a number of incompatible recommendations. At the time of writing, this may not have helped with the consultation on the DH proposals (Department of Health 2004).

We were conscious that the deliberations had been initiated by the DH in England. The Chair and Secretary of the HMRWG shared the proposals with the administrations in the home countries, Scotland, Wales and Northern Ireland, and also discussed them with representatives from the Republic of Ireland, prior to publication.

CONCLUSION: WHERE NEXT?

The reports from the HMRWG were published in September 2003 (Herbal Medicine Regulatory Working Group 2003). The HMRWG recognized from the outset that they were reports that would hopefully make a positive impact on the drive to regulate herbal medicine, but that there were no guarantees. What is clear is that they have significantly influenced the consultation by the DH (Department of Health 2004) on the proposals for the statutory regulation of herbal medicine and acupuncture. They, and the process of preparing them, have also heightened awareness within the CAM professions and amongst members of the public about the issues surrounding regulation. Lastly, the multiprofessional nature of CAM has highlighted regulatory constraints that have implications for all healthcare professionals who work across the boundaries of different regulatory bodies.

ACKNOWLEDGEMENTS

It is a pleasure to acknowledge the dedication and commitment of all members of the HMRWG without whose endeavours the reports would not have been written. In particular, thanks are due to Michael McIntyre, who taught me all I know about herbal medicine, and Amrit Ahluwalia for efficiently managing the meetings of the HMRWG. Both of these individuals put in more time than was reasonable to deliver our reports successfully.

References

Barr H 2002 Interprofessional education today, yesterday and tomorrow. Centre for Health Sciences and Practice, Learning and Teaching Support Network, London

Bristol Royal Infirmary Inquiry 2001 Report of the public inquiry into children's heart surgery at the Bristol Royal Infirmary 1984–1995. Stationery Office, London

Department of Health 1999a Making a difference: strengthening the nursing, midwifery and health visiting contribution to health and healthcare. Stationery Office, London

Department of Health 1999b Making a difference to nursing and midwifery pre-registration education. Health Service circular. Stationery Office, London

Department of Health 2000a A health service of all the talents: developing the NHS workforce consultation document on the review of workforce planning. Stationery Office, London

Department of Health 2000b The NHS plan: a plan for investment, a plan for reform. Stationery Office, London

Department of Health 2000c Meeting the challenge: a strategy for the allied health professions. Stationery Office, London

Department of Health 2001a Government response to the House of Lords Select Committee on Science and Technology's report on complementary and alternative medicine. Stationery Office, London

Department of Health 2001b Making the change. A strategy for the professions in healthcare science. Stationery Office, London

Department of Health 2001c Modernising regulation in the health professions: consultation document. Stationery Office, London

Department of Health 2004 Regulation of herbal medicine and acupuncture. Proposals for statutory regulation. Stationery Office, London

Ernst E 2003 Regulation of complementary and alternative medicine. Focus on Alternative and Complementary Therapies 8:291–292

Finch J 2000 Interprofessional education and teamworking: a view from the education providers. British Medical Journal 321:1138–1140

Freeth D, Hammick M, Koppel I et al 2002 A critical review of evaluations of interprofessional education. Centre for Health Sciences and Practice, Learning and Teaching Support Network, London

Herbal Medicine Regulatory Working Group 2003 Recommendations on the regulation of herbal practitioners in the UK including recommendations on the reform of Section 12(1) of the Medicines Act 1968. Prince of Wales's Foundation for Integrated Health, London

House of Lords' Select Committee on Science and Technology 2000 Complementary and alternative medicine. HMSO, London

Lewith G T, Breen A, Filshie J et al 2003 Complementary medicine: evidence base, competence to practice and regulation. Clinical Medicine 3:235–240

Pittilo R M, Ross F M 1998 Policies for interprofessional education: current trends in the UK. Education for Health 11:285–295.

Thomas K S, Nicoll J P, Coleman P C 2001 Use and expenditure on complementary medicine in England: a population based survey. Complementary Therapies in Medicine 9:2–11

United Kingdom Central Council for Nursing, Midwifery and Health Visiting 1999 Commission for Nursing and Midwifery Education, chair Sir Leonard Peach. UKCC, London

Herbs and herbalists:

9

professional identity and the protection of practice

Michael McIntyre

OVERVIEW

This chapter considers the history of herbal medicine, with particular reference to the use of herbal products as medicines. The use of medicines, and the relationship between the European and the national legislative powers, has been one of the more complex parts of the emergent process around statutory self-regulation. In practice, it has proved impossible to separate changes in the status of practitioners from changes in the permitted use of products. The communicating of this complex web of legislative relationships is particularly challenging.

In considering the development of legislation, the chapter examines the relationship between professional identity, professional status and professional recognition. Herbalists throughout their history have found their livelihoods under threat, often as the result of the unanticipated impact of other changes to legislation. The lack of a formal definition of the term 'herbalist' has, among other ill effects, resulted in a certain invisibility in any impact assessment of proposed new legislation. At certain times, this has proved almost catastrophic for the practitioner community.

As a result of such unanticipated threats to survival, as an unexpected side-effect of other changes to medicines law, the herbal community came to realize it had itself to play a role in the legislative process in Europe. This decision, it is argued, has mobilized the popular support of patients and raised the profile of herbalists generally, leading to a greater unity across the profession.

The chapter concludes with the proposals of the Herbal Medicine Regulatory Working Group, which it anticipates will go through on the lines recommended in their report (HMRWG 2003). Although this brings great challenges in terms of the place of herbalists among the other healthcare professions, it also offers great opportunities to educate those other professions in the benefits of herbal medicines.

BACKGROUND AND CONTEXT

Early history

For thousands of years, herbal medicine has provided the main or sometimes the only means to treat the sick amongst all peoples across the world. Indeed, until modern times, the history of herbal medicine (Western, Chinese, Ayurvedic and Tibetan) is the history of medicine itself. The herbals of Dioscorides and Galen remained among the principal medical texts throughout Asia and Europe for more than 13 centuries. The medical knowledge of the Greeks passed to the Arabs, who founded many medical schools like that in Salerno. In the twelfth century, the medicine of medieval Europe was significantly advanced by the Crusaders, who learnt herbal skills from their Arab adversaries, who passed on the knowledge of ancient Greek and Persian medicine. Christian monks were the beneficiaries of this herbal know-how; the walled gardens of medieval monasteries provided herbal medicines to treat the population of Europe. The Latin names of many medicinal plants such as *Calendula officinalis* denote that the plant was recognized as the official medicinal variety to be grown by these doctor monks.

In the reign of Henry VIII, the Herbalists' charter (Box 9.1) demonstrated, for the first time, how fiercely people would react to protect their right to have herbal treatment. This is a theme, as we shall see, that was to be repeated frequently in modern times. Indeed, public demand for herbal treatment has been the driving force to make politicians and administrators finally accept that herbal medicine must have a proper legal basis. Moreover, centuries later, the UK herbalists once again have the invaluable backing of royalty. The Prince of Wales's support for the drive towards statutory recognition, both through his Foundation for Integrated Health and directly through his personal intervention, has been hugely helpful in gaining recognition for herbalists in the twenty-first century.

The struggle for status

Throughout the latter part of the nineteenth century and the twentieth century, UK herbalists fought a constant battle to gain a secure legal basis for their right to practise and use their plant medicines. The early records of the National Association of Herbal Medicine show how herbalists were harassed and attacked by the medical establishment, which did its best to suppress and outlaw the practice of botanic medicine. In 1886, when an amendment to the Medical Acts proposed to make it illegal to practise medicine unless qualified as a doctor, the herbalists successfully campaigned against the Bill, which was subsequently withdrawn. That same year, the herbalists were also successful in preventing one of their favoured herbal remedies, *Lobelia inflata*, from being put on a new Poisons Schedule. But when, in the 1890s, the National Association sought to gain a charter that would have given their members equal status with medical practitioners, the granting of a charter was fiercely opposed by the medical establishment and the initiative foundered.

Box 9.1   The Herbalists' charter

Enacted by Henry VIII 1543 (excerpt)

By the time of Henry VIII, herbal medicine had become a lucrative business and an attempt by doctors at the King's Court to prevent others from practising medicine led to fierce resistance on the part of the population of London to preserve their right to consult whom they chose. Henry VIII gave way to public pressure, enacting the famous 'Herbalists' charter' of 1543, which gave rights to all his subjects to practise herbal medicine.

> Be it ordained, established, and enacted by Authority of this present Parliament, That at all Time from henceforth it shall be lawful to every Person being the King's subject. Having Knowledge and Experience of the Nature of Herbs, Roots, and Waters, or of the Operation of the same, by Speculation or Practice, within any part of the Realm of England, or within any other of the King's Dominions, to practice, use, and minister in and to any outward Sore, Uncome Wound, Apostemations, outward Swelling or Disease, any Herb or Herbs, Ointments, Baths, Pultess, and Emplaisters, according to their Cunning, Experience, and Knowledge in any of the Diseases, Sores, and Maladies beforesaid, and all other like to the same, or Drinks for the Stone, Strangury, or Agues, without suit, vexation, trouble, penalty, or loss of their goods . . .

Despite being opposed at every turn, herbalists were a hardy breed and, supported by their patients, continued to offer gentle and effective treatments for many conditions that were otherwise routinely treated with poisons such as mercury and arsenic. By 1923, the National Association of Medical Herbalists felt strong enough to lobby MPs for a Medical Herbalists Registration Bill, which would finally grant them safe legal status. Over 130 MPs signed up to the Private Members Bill, which miraculously enjoyed an unopposed first reading. But the hopes of the herbalists were soon dashed and the government refused to make time for the Bill to progress any further, which was hardly surprising in the light of comments by the then Chief Medical Officer of England, Sir George Newman. His response to overtures by the herbalists could hardly have been more devastating.

"The object is obviously to secure legal recognition for herbalists . . . No doubt the arguments of the promoters would be that if people wish to be treated by some kinds of herbalists, it is better to be treated by herbalists who have some kind of training than by those with none. I do not know how herbalists are trained, but it is at least doubtful whether a trained herbalist is any less dangerous than an untrained one."

(Saks 1992)

Later, the herbalists took heart at the positive advice they received from one of their foremost supporters, the MP for Jarrow, Mr R. J. Wilson, who in 1930 wrote to the National Association words of encouragement that hold good to this day. He said:

"My advice to you is to continue your education policy. Make the Medical Herbal Practitioner thorough and efficient. Make your diploma a hallmark of sound training. Eliminate the charlatan by the service that your members alone can give . . . It should be the effort, from now onwards, of every follower of the various forms of treatment outside the conventional, to enter upon research vigorously."

(Griggs 1997)

The connection between education, practice and research has been a constant theme in the history of the development of the herbal profession since this time.

The Medicines Act of 1968

But if herbalists thought that things were getting better, they were wrong. The thalidomide tragedy of the early 1960s saw the birth of thousands of children afflicted by severe physical deformities caused by this drug, which was widely prescribed as a sedative to pregnant women although it had never been properly tested. Faced with a huge public outcry about the lack of any control over drugs, the government rushed in legislation requiring the testing and licensing of all medicines. Herbal medicines were caught up in this bid to monitor and manage the marketing of drugs. The White Paper published in September 1967 proposing new legislation to control the marketing of drugs repeated the 1941 Act's prohibition on the supply of herbs by practitioners, allowing their sale only through retail outlets (Ministry of Health 1967). In fact, the White Paper sought even more draconian restrictions on herbal practice, proposing that patients could be treated only if they attended a consultation in person, so that repeat medicines could not be sent by post. Moreover, the Bill contemplated a complete embargo on dispensing medicines in the form of tinctures, fluid extracts and ointments. The Bill also proposed to restrict drastically the range of herbs used by practitioners. Taken as a whole, these measures would have closed down every herbal practitioner in the country.

A major victory was won when the proposal to give pharmacists the regulatory role to inspect herbal premises was deleted from the Bill. The proposed legislation broke new ground in that for the first time it mentioned the word 'herbalist'. Fred Fletcher Hyde, then the President of the National Institute of Medical Herbalists, later recalled that, when he requested of the Health Department that the term 'herbalist' should be defined, he was told that the definition would be provided after consultation with the pharmacists and doctors (Fletcher Hyde, personal communication 1990). Realizing that this was likely to lead to further damaging restrictions, Fred avoided mentioning the subject again and when the Medicines Act came into law the term herbalist remained undefined. This has been a significant weakness of the legislation passed in 1968, as in practice anyone may claim to be a herbalist. This matter is likely to be remedied by the statutory regulation of herbalists currently under consideration. However, before progress could be made in terms of legislation, much work was still needed to resolve the idea of a common understanding of the term 'herbalist' from the many practitioners who use herbal products.

After the 1968 Medicines Act became law, Fred Fletcher Hyde was appointed in 1970 to the 'Committee on Prescription Only Medicines', in which capacity he oversaw comments inserted into Clause 56 of the Act in which a herbalist was acknowledged as 'one who exercises his judgment as to the treatment required and accepts legal responsibility for his actions'. Fred had also helped to frame both parts of Section 12 of the Medicines' Act of 1968. Section 12(1) still provides the legal basis for herbal practitioners to treat patients following a personal consultation, critically granting an exemption from licensing for herbal prescriptions supplied on such a one-to-one basis. The importance of this piece of legislation has recently been underlined by the virtual wholesale adoption of Section 12(1) into Irish medicines law in order to protect the right of Irish herbal practitioners to prescribe for their patients. Section 12(2) gave similar exemptions from licensing for herbal products sold over the counter to the public provided these were simple plant mixtures and that the product made no health claims. Section 12(2), as we shall see, is now being replaced by the new Directive on Traditional Herbal Medicinal Products (DTHMP 2004), which became law throughout the EU in April 2004.

Box 9.2 details the background to the formation of the Council for Complementary and Alternative Medicine (CCAM).

THE EUROPEAN DIMENSION

With the benefit of hindsight, the herbalists were perhaps unwise not to forge formal links to the DH and the Medicines Control Agency (MCA) during the 1980s. As a new decade dawned, it seemed that existing UK herbal medicines legislation was threatened by European legislation. In 1992, it rapidly became clear that herbal practitioners could no longer rely on the provisions of the 1968 Medicines Act to protect their access to herbal medicines. At this time, there were great difficulties in getting herbal practitioners to come together to take a unified approach to this new threat.

There were other clear indications that herbal medicine was coming under renewed pressure. The powerful European Commission Committee on Proprietary Medicinal Products (CPMP) without any consultation, out of the blue, issued a list of what the Committee termed 'herbal drugs with serious risks, without any accepted benefit'. The list was stamped 'not acceptable for revision'. The list comprised some 30 herbs, including some such as coltsfoot (*Tussilago farfar*) and angelica root (*Angelica archangelica*), which were major remedies in use by British herbalists.

Box 9.2   The Council for Complementary and Alternative Medicine

For many herbalists, the 1980s appeared to be a time of relative security as far as their legal position was concerned. The herbal provisions of the 1968 Medicines Act provided practitioners, for the first time since 1941, with a clear legislative basis to practise herbal medicine. Herbalists maintained little contact with the government in this decade, although the manufacturers and suppliers of herbal medicines continued to work with the Medicines Control Agency (today renamed the Medicines and Healthcare Products Regulatory Agency) to review existing medicines licences for herbal products. The herbalists did, however, forge alliances with other complementary therapies to protect their interests.

In the early 1980s, the Prince of Wales as President of the British Medical Association gave a speech at a dinner to celebrate the 150th anniversary of the BMA, in which he likened modern medicine to a Leaning Tower of Pisa, often blind to the needs of the whole patient. The Prince urged conventional medics to take account of 'long neglected complementary methods of medicine' (Prince of Wales 2001). The doctors, shocked and not a little piqued to be so publicly taken to task by the Prince, launched a BMA enquiry into complementary medicine. The investigation was unashamedly biased. No complementary and alternative medicine (CAM) representative was included on the BMA committee of enquiry, nor were CAM therapies formally consulted. When the BMA report (BMA 1986) was published, it was so negative that it only attracted public ridicule. To add to the sense of injustice, a leader in the *British Medical Journal* suggested that consulting an osteopath had about as much validity as looking for answers in the entrails of birds. As a direct response to these attacks on CAM, the five main CAM therapies – herbal medicine, homeopathy, chiropractic, osteopathy and acupuncture – formed an umbrella group, the Council for Complementary and Alternative Medicine (CCAM) to fight for the interests of CAM therapies.

Public reaction to the first BMA report and the work of CCAM led to a series of ground-breaking colloquia, held with the backing and direct participation of the Prince of Wales at the Royal Society of Medicine. The colloquia engendered a fascinating debate between leading members of the CAM sector and senior doctors from within orthodox medicine. These debates, several taking place in the presence of the Prince himself, had far-reaching consequences. The BMA rethought its position on complementary medicine and published an altogether more measured and positive appraisal of CAM therapies, calling for the statutory regulation of the main CAM therapies and for doctors practising CAM to be properly trained in their chosen modality (BMA 1993). A second important outcome of the colloquia was that they provided the impetus for the launch on behalf of the Prince of Wales of the Foundation for Integrated Medicine (now renamed the Prince of Wales's Foundation for Integrated Health), an organization that was to play a major role in helping the herbal profession move towards statutory regulation throughout the 1990s and into the new millennium.

Napoleonic code

The difficulty that the European Commission had in coming to terms with the fact that in the UK there was a thriving body of professional herbalists (where practitioners in the Western herbal tradition were now practising alongside those of other traditions such as Chinese and Ayurvedic medicine) highlighted profound legislative variation within the EU. These differences have influenced the way CAM has developed in various member states. Napoleonic code, instigated by Napoleon in 1804 to determine the civil law of the French Empire, has been adapted for use by several EU member states, including France, Holland, Belgium, Italy, Portugal and Spain. A ramification of Napoleonic code, which in contrast to UK and Irish common law is not based on precedent, is that it would require specific legislation to enable CAM practitioners who are not doctors to practise medicine. In the UK and Ireland, common law has allowed willing patients to be treated by CAM practitioners without danger of being fined or sent to prison, subject in the UK to minor legal limitations (for example, non-doctor practitioners may not advertise that they treat cancer, Bright's disease, venereal disease and diabetes). In the majority of European member states, including France, Spain, Italy, Greece and Belgium, the practice of medicine except by statutorily recognized health professionals is technically illegal. This is also theoretically the situation in the Netherlands, but in practice the Dutch government does not prosecute non-doctor CAM practitioners unless there has been malpractice.

Germany has the unique *Heilpraktiker* (health practitioners) system, which licenses practitioners who are not members of recognized health professions to practise provided that they have passed an examination in basic medical knowledge and are registered. Denmark tolerates some CAM practitioners such as herbalists and homeopaths, but their practice remains a legally grey area. Non-doctor acupuncturists may practise only under the close supervision of a doctor.

It can be argued that this piecemeal approach to the way CAM may be practised throughout the EU is at variance with one of the fundamental founding principles of the European Union. This is the free movement of workers throughout the EU as laid down in the Treaty of Rome (Part 3, Title III Free Movement of Persons, Services and Capital). It seems strange that, in a market designed to allow the free movement of goods and services, non-doctor osteopaths and chiropractors who are state registered in the UK are liable to criminal prosecution if they set up in practice across the channel in France. At present, this strange anomaly is justified because each member state has the right, under the EU principle of subsidiarity, to set differing standards for professional qualifications within its own borders. Common law has encouraged the growth and development of CAM in the UK and, at the last count, no fewer than seven British universities now offer degree courses in herbal medicine. Several other university courses offer training in osteopathy and chiropractic. Yet if they are not already conventional doctors, these graduates similarly find themselves unable to work throughout most of the EU. This situation is likely to be a matter of increasingly hot debate as there is currently consultation on a new EU draft directive 'On the recognition of professional qualifications'. It is not clear what the agreed EU status of non-doctor CAM professionals will be, but the outcome is likely to be more secure for those professions that have statutory regulation in at least one member state. This is one important reason why statutory regulation of herbal practitioners in the UK may be vital for the profession's ultimate survival within the EU. Much work remains to be done within the different member states to support the development of acceptable forms of professional recognition.

The Lannoye report

In the early 1990s, these variations of approach by various member states towards CAM, and the fact that so many Europeans make use of CAM therapies, encouraged the MEP Paul Lannoye to try and advance the resources and legal status of CAM within the EU (Lannoye 1994).

As a member of the Committee of the Environment, Public Health and Consumer Protection, in 1994 he published a report on the status of complementary medicine (in subsequent versions termed 'non-conventional medicine') that made several proposals for ratification by the European Parliament. In effect, the Lannoye report sought to open the way to EU recognition of non-traditional forms of medicine (chiropractic, osteopathy, homeopathy, anthroposophical medicine, phytotherapy/herbal medicine, TCM, shiatsu and naturopathy). Amongst the report's far-reaching proposals were provisions for recognition and harmonization of CAM qualifications and training throughout the EU. In addition, it called for the inclusion of certain alternative medical disciplines in the teaching of conventional medicine, and the inclusion in the European pharmacopoeia of the full range of supplements and herbal products used as non-conventional medicines so as to guarantee the quality and safety of such products. Lannoye also petitioned the Commission to fund a full research programme into the efficacy of CAM treatments and to draft a directive to guarantee CAM practitioners the freedom to provide their services throughout the EU and to access the therapeutic products they need in the exercise of their profession.

Unsurprisingly, the Lannoye report met with fierce opposition from the medical and pharmaceutical lobby. The first report was adopted by the Committee on the Environment, Public Health and Consumer Protection but was filibustered so that it ran out of time when it was debated in the European Parliament. Determined to succeed, Lannoye tried again with a second report in 1996. This too reached the European Parliament where it met a barrage of amendments that so reduced its scope that Lannoye insisted that his name be removed from the final version. In effect all that remained of the original report, ratified by the European Parliament as the 'Collins resolution' in 1997, was its call on the Commission to research the CAM sector. Despite the personal commitment of such individuals as Paul Lannoye, it continues to be difficult to get legislative time, at both EU and member state level, to address the issues of the professional identity of herbal practitioners, including the mobility of qualified individuals.

The European Herbal Practitioners Association

In 1993, a group of leading practitioners decided to launch a new umbrella organization that would comprise registers of herbalists of all traditions in the United Kingdom and Europe. The new organization was called the European Herbal Practitioners Association (EHPA). The EHPA was founded to represent the interests of herbalists in the UK and Europe and to unify the profession in order to begin talks with the government in the UK (and possibly other member states) about the recognition of herbal practitioners and, in addition, to safeguard access to herbal medicines.

In the autumn of 1994 the MCA, in anticipation of the launch of the Single Market in pharmaceutical products and the establishment of the new European Medicines Evaluation Agency (EMEA), published a consultation document (MLX 206). This announced their plans to harmonize the UK Medicines Act of 1968 with the main European Medicines Directive (then called Directive 65/65 EEC). The effect of this would be to annul those sections of the UK 1968 Medicines Act (Section 12 and 36) that allowed herbal medicines to be prescribed and sold without a medicines licence. Since herbs cannot be patented like drugs, the cost of licensing them as medicines would be prohibitive. Consequently, as the majority of herbal products had no licences, all UK herbal suppliers and practitioners were threatened with being driven out of business on 1 January 1995 when the new EU regulations came into force. Herbal practitioners who relied on their suppliers for their herbs, tinctures, pills and ointments would also effectively be unable to practice. The UK herbal community stared disaster in the face.

The government was adamant that there was nothing that could be done so, finally, the herbal community went public with the story. Once again, as in 1967, a nationwide public campaign on behalf of herbal medicine was launched. The matter was made worse for the government since the first degree course in herbal medicine had just been validated at Middlesex University. The UK MCA was deluged with over a hundred thousand outraged letters from the public. MPs and MEPs were similarly showered with angry letters from their constituents. Government lawyers immediately came up with an ingenious piece of legal 'sticking plaster' to patch over the troublesome phrase within the main medicines law that said that 'industrially produced' medicines must be licensed (or in Euro-terminology hold a marketing authorization), declaring that herbal medicines were 'traditionally rather than industrially produced'. As a result the government lawyers were pleased to announce that herbal medicines were not after all subject to EU medicines legislation (Directive 65/65 EEC) and so did not require a licence. The solution may have been all smoke and mirrors, but for the time being the crisis was over.

The Irish question

A similar herbal uproar occurred in Ireland in 1999, when the Irish Medicines Board (IMB) suddenly, and without consultation, declared that St John's wort (*Hypericum perforatum*) and a number of other well-known herbal remedies were to be prescription-only medicines from 1 January 2000. Consequently, the new Irish legislation amounted to a ban on these herbs since no licensed versions of them existed on the Irish market. The IMB's ruling caused similar outrage amongst the Irish public to that in 1994 in the UK, and the Irish Health Minister was forced to intervene on behalf of Irish herbalists to enable practitioners to continue to use the herbs that had been designated prescription only. These two herbal crises in the UK and in Ireland had similar outcomes. Both the UK authorities and their Irish counterparts were compelled to give the status of herbal medicine high priority and both the MCA and IMB began working on new legislation to underpin the supply of herbal medicines. In both cases, the EHPA played a major role in campaigning on behalf of the herbal profession.

In search of a European directive on herbal medicine

The EHPA wasted no time in seeking more long-term solutions. A position paper entitled 'Alternative licensing for herbal medicine-like products in the European Union' was drafted. This paper called for a new directive allowing herbs on to the European market without the need for a full market authorization (i.e. licence) so long as these herbal medicines could demonstrate safe traditional use.

Fortunately, the EHPA were not alone in seeking a pan-European solution. The UK MCA was also pressing the European Commission for a new herbal directive and, after consulting with UK herbalists and manufacturers, came up with a draft proposal, which it put to the Commission and other member states. After the St John's wort Irish herb crisis detailed above, the IMB supported the UK initiative.

In 1999 the European Commission received a report on the current status of herbal medicines throughout Europe. One of the key findings of this report was that most member states were failing to apply EU medicines legislation to herbal medicines because, in reality, the law had proved unworkable. The report made plain the legislative impasse faced by plant medicine suppliers, who could never recoup the huge sums of money required to license a medicine as their products could not be patented. As a result the Commission itself moved to introduce specific EU legislation for herbal products based on the proposals first put forward by the UK MCA.

After several drafts, consultations and debates in Brussels and elsewhere, the Directive on Traditional Herbal Medicinal Products (DTHMP 2004) finally became law throughout the European Union in April 2004. This landmark legislation allows for over-the-counter herbal products to be marketed for self-limiting minor ailments with a traditional medicinal licence produced under Good Manufacturing Practice (GMP). To qualify for a DTHMP licence, the herbs in the product should demonstrate 30 years' continuous safe use. In the case of herbal medicines originating outside the EU, evidence of 15 years of the required total of 30 years of safe use must be demonstrated within the EU to qualify for a DTHMP licence. DTHMP products are required to carry limited medical claims and may include a limited range of vitamins and minerals. In the UK, the DTHMP licensing system will be implemented over the next 7 years and will replace the exemption from licensing granted by Section 12(2) of the 1968 Medicines Act, which will become obsolete in time.

In the context of this directive, it is important to note specifically the protections offered to herbal medicines originating outside the EU. It is likely that, without the intervention of the EHPA, many Chinese and Ayurvedic products would have been excluded from the legislation. This is one example of the protection that can be offered by a unified profession.

DEVELOPMENTS IN THE UK STATUTORY REGULATION OF HERBALISTS

The EHPA was not only concerned with pursuing a new European directive on herbal medicines. Shortly after its launch, in 1994, it approached the UK DH asking to discuss the statutory regulation of herbal practitioners, which would afford herbal practitioners legal status in the UK. In particular, it was clear that Section 12(1) of the 1968 Medicines Act, which conferred exemptions from licensing for herbal medicines prescribed by practitioners directly to their patients on a on-to-one basis, was thoroughly inadequate. As it contained no definition of the term herbalist, there were no safeguards to determine who might prescribe powerful herbs that had been put on a Schedule in SI 2130 (a statutory instrument of the 1968 Medicines Act). The osteopaths and the chiropractors had recently achieved statutory regulation and the DH was open to the idea that the herbalists might be next in line.

The EHPA was advised by civil servants at the Department of Health (DH) to draw together practitioners of all traditions using herbs in the UK. The EHPA had already begun this process – a task made significantly easier by the unity of purpose experienced by the herbal sector during the struggle with the UK government in 1994 over the legal basis of herbal supplies. From 1995 onwards, it was clear that the MCA was as keen as the DH itself on herbalists becoming statutorily regulated, as this would allow the agency to identify those individuals prescribing herbs on a one-to-one basis. The MCA was understandably concerned at reports about the misidentification, adulteration, contamination and inadequate quality control of herbs, particularly in the Chinese herbal and Ayurvedic sectors. A scandalous case of herbal poisoning had come to light in Belgium in the early 1990s, where doctors had prescribed a 'herbal' slimming pill comprising a misidentified Chinese herb, *Aristolochia manchuriensis*, deadly nightshade, amphetamine and acetazolamide, a diuretic. This mixture proved deadly for over 200 women in Belgium and research revealed that aristolochic acid was the main toxin involved, causing severe kidney damage. Investigations by the MCA exposed the fact that herbs of the *Aristolochia* family had also been mistakenly sold in the UK. The EHPA and its constituent organizations worked closely with the MCA to rectify the situation. The need for better herbal regulation was all the more evident in the light of this and other herbal safety issues that have arisen subsequently.

The House of Lords Select Committee report and the Government response

By 1999, the EHPA had become the main umbrella organization, representing herbal practitioners in negotiation with the European Commission and the UK MCA and DH. Leading members of the EHPA toured the country talking to practitioners about statutory regulation. The EHPA disseminated information about its work via its website and occasional newsletter, *Frankincense*.

That year, the House of Lords Committee on Science and Technology decided to enquire into and report on complementary medicine. The EHPA made a written and personal submission to the Select Committee, advocating that herbal practitioners should be statutorily regulated and measures taken to ensure the quality and safety of herbal medicines. Yvette Cooper, Parliamentary Under-Secretary of State for Health, also gave evidence to the Select Committee, saying that the government had identified herbal medicine and acupuncture as specific therapies it would like to see achieve statutory regulation (House of Lords 2000).

When the Select Committee published its seminal report in November 2000, it specifically identified herbal medicine as posing particular challenges for public health and recommended that acupuncture and herbal practitioners should be statutorily regulated. In addition, it called for herbal medicines to have assured quality and safety. The Select Committee noted that effective regulation of practitioners would safeguard the public from poorly trained and incompetent practitioners. It would identify practitioners suitably qualified to use a range of potent herbal remedies that are not appropriate for OTC sale. In March 2001, the DH responded to the Select Committee report expressing the view that herbal practitioners and acupuncturists should work towards statutory regulation under the Health Act of 1999 (Government response 2001). This Act provided a fast-track route to statutory regulation, no longer relying, as had been the case for osteopaths and chiropractors, on an expensive and cumbersome primary legislation to achieve the same end. The DH recommended that, taking account of public health risks posed by the herbal and acupuncture sectors, statutory regulation of acupuncturists and herbalists should be implemented as soon as possible.

The launch of the Herbal Medicine Regulatory Working Group

On 30 December 2001, the *Sunday Times* ran a major news story in which it declared that the Secretary of State for Health, Alan Milburn, wanted complementary practitioners to be licensed to work under contract to the NHS, using approved medicines and treatments. The report said that Milburn's decision followed research by an all-party Lords' committee, which concluded that some herbal remedies were as effective as conventional medicines and in some cases worked better than antibiotics.

The story was inaccurate in several respects, but the paper did correctly report that the government had appointed Professor Mike Pittilo, Pro-Vice Chancellor of the University of Hertfordshire, as an independent Chair to head up a working group to look into the statutory regulation of herbalists. The Herbal Medicine Regulatory Working Group (HMRWG) was launched the following day, on 1 January 2002, with the backing of three stakeholders: the DH, the Prince of Wales's Foundation for Integrated Health (PoWFIH) and the EHPA.

The HMRWG had two main terms of reference. First, it was asked to produce a report examining the options for successful statutory regulation of the herbal profession as a whole to form the basis of wider consultation by the government, and subsequently for legislation to enable the statutory regulation of herbalists. Secondly, it was asked to review Section 12(1) of the Medicines Act of 1968 (concerning one-to-one prescription by practitioners) to make recommendations for assuring the quality and safety of herbal remedies supplied under this piece of legislation. It should be noted that because the 12(1) type of prescription of herbs takes place on a one-to-one basis, and remedies are prescribed individually, these herbal medicines are technically not placed on the European market as products and so remain subject to UK law (Section 12(1) of the 1968 Medicines Act) rather than to the main European medicines directive – now renamed 2001/83/EC. The complexity of medicines law, and the interrelationship between medicines law and practitioner status, is one of the greatest barriers to communication with the community of practitioners about the case for statutory self-regulation.

The Acupuncture Regulatory Working Group (ARWG) was launched a few weeks later, independently chaired by Lord Chan of Oxton, with a number of acupuncture stakeholders as well as the DH and PoWFIH. It followed similar terms of reference regarding the statutory regulation of acupuncturists (ARWG 2003).

Recommendations from the HMRWG

The HMRWG met regularly over a period of 18 months. The Committee surveyed the scope of herbal practice in the UK and published its findings in September 2003 (HMRWG 2003). It found that there were approximately 1300 herbal medicine practitioners who are members of voluntary registers in the UK. It noted that the size of these registers was approximately equal for the traditions of Western herbal medicine and Chinese herbal medicine. The numbers of practitioners of Ayurvedic and Tibetan medicine were small by comparison. The HMRWG report had the support of all the main UK herbal registers except for one of the three UK Ayurvedic groups, which disassociated itself from the agreed common-core curriculum (Box 9.3), despite the fact that this curriculum had the backing of the Department of the Indian Systems of Medicine (Chapter 8).

Box 9.3   Core curriculum and accreditation

In 1994, the EHPA began working on a core curriculum to be held in common by all the professional herbal registers that had come together under its banner. The EHPA included Western herbal professional associations, a Chinese herbal association and a TCM association as well as a Tibetan and Ayurvedic association. All the associations in the EHPA agreed that a good standard of training in Western biomedicine was essential for safe practice and that tradition-specific modules should be devised for each of the traditions represented within the EHPA. In addition, the EHPA agreed a position paper on continuing professional development for qualified practitioners of herbal medicine. Representatives from other member states (most importantly Ireland and Denmark) were involved in the development of the curriculum for entry and the proposals for continuing professional development. However, to date, no other country in Europe outside the UK and Ireland has yet agreed to adopt a common approach to education and training nationally, across all the practitioner bodies and training schools.

The HMRWG proposed the establishment of a council to have responsibility for establishing and maintaining a register of practitioners competent to prescribe and use herbal medicines. Such a council would determine the minimum level of education and training, along with levels of competence required for registration. In addition, the HMRWG recommended that the current EHPA Accreditation Board should in due course be managed by the new council and that the council should have four statutory committees, paralleling those of other statutory healthcare councils. Statutory registration would confer on registered practitioners the right to use a protected title, which would identify competence in a particular tradition(s).

The HMRWG also made other recommendations concerning the prescription of herbal medicines on a one-to-one basis (from practitioner to patient). Reform of the relevant sections of the Medicines Act of 1968 would allow registered practitioners access to potent herbal remedies that would otherwise be restricted from OTC sale direct to the public. It would also allow specific herbal formulations to be made up under Good Manufacturing Practice to the herbalist's specification. This would be possible under an exemption from licensing granted to the 'authorized health professionals' by the main EU Medicines Directive (2001/83/EC), so dispensing with the need for prohibitively expensive medicines licences for these industrially produced products. The HMRWG expressed the view that all those currently supplying unlicensed herbal medicines on a one-to-one basis should probably eventually be brought under the control of the statutory council. The HMRWG also suggested that registered herbal practitioners should be permitted to use traditional medicines of non-plant origin provided these remedies could demonstrate a history of safe use and were subject to required quality standards. Both these latter two recommendations are problematic in terms of clear definitions about their scope.

The Department of Health consultation document and MLX 299

On 2 March 2004, the DH and the Medicines and Healthcare products Regulatory Agency (MHRA) simultaneously published two consultation documents, the 'Regulation of herbal medicine and acupuncture' (Department of Health 2004) and MLX 299, 'Proposals for the reform of the regulation of unlicensed herbal remedies in the United Kingdom made up to meet the needs of individual patients' (MHRA 2004).

The consultation period on these two documents closed on 7 June 2004 and by autumn 2004 the DH expected to prepare a Draft Order under Section 60 of the Health Act of 1999. This was to be published subsequently as a further consultation document, probably in early 2005, together with a narrative text explaining the Draft Order. The consultation period was to last a further 3 months, after which an Order is expected to be laid before, and debated by, the UK Parliament and the Scottish Parliament.

At the time of writing, it is expected that these two reports will set in train a process leading to the establishment of a new regulatory body (probably sometime in 2006), after which there will be a 2-year transitional period during which practitioners currently in practice can be admitted to the Register. During this period, the MHRA will be following a similar pathway, with the publication of a Draft Order for the reform of Section 12(1) of the 1968 Medicines Act, which will in turn lead an Order set before the Parliaments in Westminster and Edinburgh. In addition to consulting the public and other health professionals, the MHRA will also be seeking the opinion of the Medicines Commission and the Committee on the Safety of Medicines.

The DH takes a definite position on some of the issues where there were different views expressed by the HMRWG (2003) and ARWG (2003) reports. On the question of the type of regulatory body that should be established, the DH consultation document (2004) comes down firmly on the side of the establishment of a shared CAM Council for herbal medicine and acupuncture (Section 22). The DH's consultation document also expressed a definite view on the position of practitioners who are already regulated. The DH declares itself not in favour of the scheme suggested by the ARWG, whereby doctors, nurses and physiotherapists also practising acupuncture who are already statutorily registered should have the possibility of also having their names on the new regulatory body's register (in effect creating a working distinction between the regulatory functions of the new council and its registering functions) (ARWG 2003). Instead, the DH says that it prefers those already registered to remain with their primary register, recommending that the new council should provide professional leadership to all healthcare professions in respect of standards for the practice of herbal medicine and acupuncture (DH 2004, Section 49). It needs to be said that all the issues raised by the DH document are, at the time of writing, still a matter of consultation and it remains to be seen how these questions will be resolved. Small though the community of herbalists is, the ramifications of the report of the HMRWG (2003) are proving to impact on very large numbers of other kinds of professional. This means in practice that decisions on the future of herbalists are coming to be inextricably linked with wider changes in healthcare professional identity. Some argue that the agenda for complementary medicine, at least, is being disproportionally influenced by herbalists and the need to regulate better for herbal medicine products.

CONCLUSION: THE GREENING OF MEDICINE

This is a story of centuries of struggle by the herbal profession in the United Kingdom to achieve legislative security and status for both practitioners and the medicines they use. At long last, it seems that the government in the UK, and to some extent in the European Commission, is willing to provide a comprehensive legal framework to support the delivery of herbal medicine in the UK and Europe. The reason for this change of attitude on the part of the authorities is easy to see. On the one hand, there is the increasing popularity of herbal treatment as an alternative or complement to conventional medicine. This popular appeal has finally convinced the government and the medical establishment to make legislative room for this ancient form of medicine. On the other hand, the recent extraordinary growth of herbal medicine undoubtedly has put pressure on the powers that be to safeguard the public from inadequate herbal practice and poor quality herbal medicines. It is very likely that, once the new legal framework is in place, the added security it provides in terms of quality and safety will see the use and popularity of herbal medicine grow by leaps and bounds. This will be underpinned, one hopes, by well-designed research to assess the efficacy of herbal treatment for a wide range of common complaints. Although herbal practitioners will undoubtedly remain the herbal medicine experts, I predict that it will not be too long before many doctors will also find themselves routinely using gentle plant medicines as a remedy of choice in place of conventional drugs: chamomile to help you to sleep, St John's wort for mild depression, black cohosh for hot flushes, ginseng for exhaustion, echinacea and garlic for colds, gingko for poor circulation? The drug companies may not like it, but I have no doubt the patients will.

References

Acupuncture Regulatory Working Group 2003 The statutory regulation of the acupuncture profession. Prince of Wales's Foundation for Integrated Health, London

British Medical Association 1986 Alternative therapy: report of the Board of Science and Education. British Medical Association, London

British Medical Association 1993 Complementary medicine: new approaches to good practice. Oxford University Press, Oxford

Department of Health 2004 Regulation of herbal medicine and acupuncture: proposals for statutory regulation. Stationery Office, London

DTHMP 2004 The traditional herbal medicinal products directive, 2004/24/EC. Official Journal of the European Union 30 April, Brussels

Government response to the House of Lords Select Committee on Science and Technology's report on complementary and alternative medicine, March 2001. Stationery Office, London

Griggs B 1997 The new green pharmacy: the story of Western herbal medicine. Vermilion, London

Herbal Medicine Regulatory Working Group 2003 Recommendations on the regulation of herbal practitioners in the UK. Prince of Wales's Foundation for Integrated Health, London

House of Lords' Select Committee on Science and Technology 2000 Complementary and alternative medicine, 6th report. Stationery Office, London

Lannoye, P 1994 DOC – EN/RR/251/251535PE208.336, later re-issued, including (1997) PE216.0666/fin. Stationery Office, London

Medicines and Health Products Regulatory Agency 2004 MLX 299: Proposals for the reform of the regulation of unlicensed herbal remedies in the United Kingdom made up to meet the needs of individual patients. Stationery Office, London

Ministry of Health 1967 Forthcoming legislation on the safety, quality and description of drugs and medicines. Stationery Office, London

Prince of Wales 2001 The best of both worlds – personal views. British Medical Journal 322:181

Saks, M (ed) 1992 Alternative medicine in Britain. Clarendon Press, Oxford

Further reading

The Medicines for Human Use (Marketing Authorisations, Pharmacovigilance and Related Matters) Regulations 1994. Stationery Office, London

Culture and knowledge in the development of Traditional Chinese Medicine

10

Nick Lampert

OVERVIEW

This chapter offers an introduction to some of the cultural difficulties experienced by those from non-Western traditions in adapting to the norms of the UK structures of health and education. It has been widely accepted within the UK Chinese medicine community that statutory regulation is desirable for Chinese herbal medicine and for acupuncture. This will provide reassurance to the public that practitioners are suitably qualified to practise, are up to date with new developments, and bound by strict ethical rules. It also offers the opportunity for practitioners to enter into constructive dialogue with other health professionals, with the longer-term prospect of a closer working relationship with the NHS.

At the same time, practitioners are anxious to ensure that inclusion within a statutory framework will not compromise the unique contribution that the tradition can make to healthcare. Inclusion within such a framework raises a number of questions about the nature of tradition and knowledge, which are the focus of the present chapter. These questions will be discussed with reference to Chinese medicine, but they are relevant to other traditions that have a presence in the UK, including Ayurveda, Kampo and Tibetan medicine, and indeed to Western herbal medicine itself.

The chapter will look at:

- the report of the House of Lords Committee on Complementary and Alternative Medicine, and the Government response to it
- the choice between biomedical dominance and medical pluralism
- traditional and pharmacological knowledge in relation to the materia medica
- questions of research design in clinical trials
- the importance of dialogue between conventional and non-conventional medicine
- the question of translation from one medical discourse to another.

BACKGROUND: THE REPORT OF THE HOUSE OF LORDS SCIENCE AND TECHNOLOGY COMMITTEE

In its report on complementary and alternative medicine (CAM) in November 2000, the House of Lords Science and Technology Committee drew up a categorization of CAM therapies that caused some consternation amongst practitioners of non-Western traditions of medicine, in particular the Chinese and Ayurvedic traditions. The report identified three groups (House of Lords 2000). The first comprised the 'big five' disciplines of osteopathy, chiropractic, acupuncture, herbal medicine and homeopathy, each of which were seen as having an 'individual diagnostic approach'. The second group contained therapies that are 'most often used to complement conventional medicine and do not purport to embrace diagnostic skills', including, for example, aromatherapy, the Alexander technique, bodywork therapies including massage, counselling and stress therapy. The third group included:

"those other disciplines which purport to offer diagnostic information as well as treatment and which, in general, favour a philosophical approach and are indifferent to the scientific principles of conventional medicine."

(House of Lords Select Committee 2000)

This group in turn was divided into two subcategories, namely: 'long-established and traditional systems of healthcare such as Ayurvedic medicine and Traditional Chinese Medicine' and 'other alternative disciplines which lack any credible evidence base such as crystal therapy, iridology, radionics, dowsing and kinesiology'.

Osteopathy and chiropractic were already under statutory regulation. The report judged that acupuncture and herbal medicine, and possibly non-medical homeopathy, had also reached a stage where it would be of benefit both to patients and to practitioners if they were to be included within a statutory framework. Beyond the need to protect the public against the risks of incompetent practice, this conclusion was based on:

- the nature of the therapy's diagnostic claims
- the extent of its evidence base.

In relation to diagnosis, the report concluded that 'diagnostic procedures must be reliable and reproducible and more attention must be paid to whether CAM diagnostic procedures ... have been scientifically validated'. In relation to the efficacy of treatment the conclusion was that:

"while the question of efficacy was not included in our initial terms of reference, in the absence of a credible evidence base it is our opinion that the therapies listed in our Group 3 cannot be supported unless and until convincing research evidence of efficacy based upon the results of well-conducted trials can be produced. Such evidence must be capable of showing that the effects of any therapeutic discipline are superior to those of the placebo effect."

(House of Lords 2000)

The Lords' report provided a thorough and comprehensive survey of the state of many CAM therapies in the UK, with numerous useful recommendations relating to regulation, training and research. However, the grouping of therapies raised fundamental issues about the way in which the value of therapies was being assessed. On one level, the report was much criticized by herbalists for its failure to consider the research evidence that was available in the fields of Chinese and Ayurvedic medicine. On another level, and of deeper concern, was the suggestion that only those therapies that shared the framework of Western biomedicine (including, by inference, Western 'scientific' herbalism and acupuncture) could be taken seriously. This position was not consistently applied, since homeopathy was placed in the first group, although the diagnostic models and the physiological mechanisms of homeopathy remain quite mysterious from a conventional point of view, and homeopathy has been regularly rejected on account of its lack of scientific credibility. This raised the suspicion that, in the eyes of the report, a therapy could become respectable so long as it was practised by doctors. But, whatever the reason for the inconsistency, the wider issue was the relationship between Western biomedical thinking and other models of health and disease.

In its response to the report, published in March 2001, the government was in agreement with most of the recommendations. It did, however, distance itself from the view that traditional systems of medicine were unworthy of support:

"the Government considers that, for the purposes of professional self-regulation, those aspects of the traditional therapies ... which include the use of herbal remedies could come together within a federal grouping of therapies in Group 1 under the general heading of herbal medicine, while still retaining their individual identities and traditions. It may also be possible to bring within Group 1 those aspects of traditional therapies which practise acupuncture."

(Government response March 2001).

As a result of this stance, the regulatory working group that was set up for herbal medicine in January 2002 included representatives from Chinese medicine and Ayurveda as well as from Western herbal medicine. It was accepted from the start that a statutory structure would include practitioners from these traditions, and from other traditions as appropriate. Alongside essential training in biomedical sciences, a statutory body would thus set educational standards for forms of medicine that, in key respects, were strikingly different from biomedicine, advised by committees that would support the knowledge base of each tradition. The recommendations of the group were published in September 2003 (Herbal Medicine Regulatory Working Group 2003), alongside the recommendations of a parallel regulatory working group for acupuncture (Acupuncture Regulatory Working Group 2003). These formed the basis of a subsequent Department of Health consultation document on the statutory regulation of herbal medicine and acupuncture (Department of Health 2004). This document was in particular welcomed within the Chinese medicine community, because it acknowledged the integral nature of Chinese medicine practice (comprising herbal medicine and acupuncture), and proposed the adoption of Traditional Chinese Medicine as a statutory title. At the time of writing, it is expected that legislation to regulate herbal medicine and acupuncture will come on to the UK statute book in 2006, though the precise form that this will take is not yet clear.

BIOMEDICAL DOMINANCE OR MEDICAL PLURALISM?

The Government response to the House of Lords report, and the manner in which the Herbal Medicine Regulatory Working Group (HMRWG) was constituted, gave encouragement to those traditions that felt they had been given short shrift within the House of Lords report itself. However, the movement towards statutory regulation has raised fears among practitioners that herbal medicine may increasingly be judged in accordance with biomedical concepts and criteria, with a consequent loss of autonomy and ability to make its specific contribution to healthcare.

The associations representing the herbal traditions are committed to protecting patients through publicly recognized standards of competence and ethical practice, to the development of a stronger research base and to a closer relationship with the NHS. At the same time they seek to establish a framework of regulation in which a variety of traditions, with their distinctive language of description, diagnosis and treatment, would find a legitimate place.

In brief, the issue is how to retain the vitality of the herbal traditions while supporting the goal of integrated healthcare. It is a question of what is meant by 'integration'. If it is understood as absorption by biomedicine, then most practitioners of herbal medicine will find the price too high. If, by contrast, integration means a mutual respect for different forms of diagnosis and treatment, or a willingness to offer patients a range of treatments including herbal medicines or other complementary therapies, then it will be widely welcomed by herbalists and other CAM therapists.

Two perspectives on integration are set out in Box 10.1. One is a statement by the head of the United States National Center for Complementary and Alternative Medicine, invited to predict the state of CAM therapies in 2020. The other is taken from an editorial on complementary medicine in the *British Medical Journal*.

In one sense, the statement by Straus expresses a noble ideal, in which all therapies are welcomed so long as they can demonstrate efficacy and a rational foundation. But an integrated medicine that '[incorporates CAM therapies] into conventional medical education and practice' represents the hegemony of a single model. By contrast, the statement by Rees & Weil comes closer to a pluralist concept of medicine, recognizing different perspectives on health and disease, though even here the reference to 'solidly orthodox treatments' does not quite suggest recognition of different diagnostic models.

Box 10.1   Two perspectives on integration

Stephen E Straus, Head of the US National Center for Complementary and Alternative Medicine (in Goldsmith 1999):

As a result of rigorous scientific investigation, several therapeutic and preventive modalities currently deemed elements of complementary and alternative medicine will have proven effective. Therefore, by 2020, these interventions will have been incorporated into conventional medical education and practice, and the term 'complementary and alternative medicine' will be superseded by the concept of 'integrative medicine'.

The biological and pharmacological basis for effectiveness of selected herbal and nutritional supplements will be clarified, leading to their standardization and to the rational design of yet more potent congeners. Advances in neurobiology will elucidate mechanisms underlying ancient practices such as acupuncture and meditation, as well as the phenomenon of 'the placebo effect'.

Other modalities will have proven unsafe or ineffective, and an informed public will have rejected them.

The field of integrative medicine will be seen as providing novel insights and tools for human health, and not as a source of intellectual and philosophical tension that insinuates itself between and among practitioners of the healing arts and their patients . . .

Lesley Rees and Andrew Weil, Editorial in the *British Medical Journal* (Rees & Weil 2001):

Integrated medicine (or integrative medicine as it is referred to in the United States) is practising medicine in a way that selectively incorporates elements of complementary and alternative medicine into comprehensive treatment plans alongside solidly orthodox methods of diagnosis and treatment. . .

Integrated medicine is not simply a synonym for complementary medicine. Complementary medicine refers to treatments that may be used as adjuncts to conventional treatment . . . Integrated medicine has a larger meaning and mission, its focus being on health and healing rather than disease and treatment. It views patients as whole people with minds and spirits as well as bodies and includes these dimensions into diagnosis and treatment. It also involves patients and doctors working to maintain health by paying attention to lifestyle factors such as diet, exercise, quality of rest and sleep, and the nature of relationships.

. . . Integrated medicine is not just about teaching doctors to use herbs instead of drugs. It is about restoring core values which have been eroded by social and economic forces. Integrated medicine is good medicine, and its success will be signalled by dropping the adjective.

The following account will look at the thinking that underlies the pursuit of an ideal of medical pluralism. It envisages the coexistence of different medical traditions, each with a distinctive discourse, in a context of openness and dialogue rather than closure and monologue. It will consider:

- the inability of any single medical model to encompass the whole clinical reality
- the importance of traditional understanding and usage of the materia medica, alongside pharmacological analysis
- the need for flexibility in research design in assessing the efficacy of herbal medicine
- the need for communication between the herbal traditions and orthodox medicine
- the question whether, in the pursuit of such communication, a translation of concepts from one medical discourse to another is possible.

NO SINGLE MODEL ENCOMPASSES THE WHOLE REALITY

A pluralistic conception of health provision is based on the understanding that no single model of health and disease can encompass clinical reality as a whole. Any form of description is a partial representation of phenomena and whatever language of description is used, whether verbal or mathematical, a process of filtering and construction is involved (Flower, unpublished essay, 2003). A definition of research, for example, as 'the systematic and rigorous process of enquiry which aims to describe phenomena and to develop and test explanatory concepts and theories' (Bowling 2002), takes 'description' as unproblematic. Yet observers begin with their own notions of reality, their own personal and corporate agendas and conceptual frameworks. These condition what is seen and what remains unseen (Flower 2003).

Awareness of the limited nature of any model of clinical reality need not lead to a relativism in which 'anything goes'. But it is a necessary starting point for an appreciation of the insights that Chinese medicine has to offer. This was well illustrated in a round-table discussion published in the journal of the Register of Chinese Herbal Medicine (Protecting the Chinese medicine tradition, Buck 2002, Wright 2002) (Box 10.2).

THE MATERIA MEDICA

A pluralistic approach to medical models also means taking on board the traditional understanding of the properties of the materia medica (for details see Chapter 3) The description of those properties is based upon observed effects over a very long history, and provides essential tools for clinical practice. As noted in Chapter 3, the art of treatment with Chinese herbal medicine is to choose a formula that matches the pattern of disharmony of the individual, and to modify the formula in order to accommodate changes in

Box 10.2   Chinese medicine and biomedicine

Charles Buck (practitioner of Chinese medicine), in a round-table discussion on Chinese medicine and biomedicine:

The question is how do we explain the fact that we can use alternate models to describe the same thing, the human body in health and disease, and for both to remain valid. The crux of the issue is that Chinese medicine aims to describe clinical functionality and Western medicine aims to use technology to describe substance. When I explain this to a medically scientific audience I start with a slide of a series of chemicals: calcium phosphate, carbohydrates, fatty acids, etc and ask 'what is this?'. Usually there are mumblings about it being the constituents of the human body. The next slide is of Vermeer's 'Lady with a Pearl Earring'. Yes, I say, that was a valid chemical analysis of the picture, one that may be useful in verifying the authenticity of the painting, but you could also take it to a Sotheby's expert whose language would be in terms of colour, composition, content and brush strokes. Both are valid descriptions and both could be used to authenticate the painting, but the language is aiming to describe something different, different qualities are measured.

Some diseases are the result of a single chemical or pathological change. These are the diseases most easily tackled by biomedicine. Many other illnesses involve a tidal shift of thousands of variables, this is not easily amenable to simple chemical analysis. This is why the clinically derived label 'Spleen Deficiency' is so valuable. It is a summary of a global change, one that empirical experiment has found can be altered. My argument against the chemist is that the body is impossibly complex, not always amenable to reductionism.

... This is the problem with biomedicine. It doesn't have a language of clinical reality, or one that can understand and describe what really happens to actual people, in health and disease. Chinese medicine is the medicine of systematic clinical experience par excellence.

(Buck 2002)

Mark Wright (practitioner of Chinese medicine), in the same round-table discussion:

The biomedical model has a lot in its favour, and if I am run over and mangled by a bus, I won't be looking for a herbalist, I will be jolly glad of biomedicine. But the Chinese medicine model also has a great deal in its favour. I use the metaphor of the toolbox. A spanner is excellent for adjusting nuts and bolts. A screwdriver is excellent for adjusting screws. A hammer is great for hammering in nails. We could use a large screwdriver for hammering in nails, but it is not well suited. In practice, what we do is choose the right tool for the job. Sometimes a screwdriver and a spanner

---

Box 10.2   (Continued)

work best together. Yet we do not seek to understand or deploy the screwdriver in the spanner's terms, or vice versa.

Sometimes one is better, sometimes another, and at other times they work together each in their own separate ways. The problem is that whereas we practice Chinese medicine and happily acknowledge that the biomedical model is good within certain limitations, the biomedical practitioners do not reciprocate. I would always seek to speak to medics in their own terms so far as possible in the hopes that, finally, they may meet us halfway. The only sad thing is the reluctance of the biomedical fraternity to meet us in an equable and open-minded fashion.

(Wright 2002)

---

the course of treatment. A mastery of this process requires a thorough under-standing of the properties of the materia medica as described in the tradition, as well as the development of sophisticated diagnostic skills.

This form of understanding does not exclude the application of pharma-cological knowledge, and there is a large and growing body of pharmacological research on Chinese medicinal herbs (exemplified by Amano et al 1996, Chang et al 1997, Oishi et al 1998, Suzuki et al 1997, Yoshida et al 1997). Such research indicates that traditional uses of plant remedies and the known physiological activity of plant constituents often coincide. However, herbal medicine is pharmacologically far more complex than pharmaceutical medi-cine, which seeks a narrow target with one or very few active ingredients. In contrast, herbal medicine relies on a multiplicity of constituents, some of which may have a synergistic or buffering effect. The complexity becomes greater still when ingredients are combined – as typically occurs in Chinese medicine – so as to accommodate flexibly the characteristics of individual patients. This complexity is a virtue, but becomes a stumbling block for phar-maceutical companies looking for isolated active ingredients in herbal medi-cines that could be standardized and marketed.

It is undoubtedly through their chemical constituents that herbal medicines exert their effects. But, given the complexity of the conditions treated and the substances used, clinical practice cannot be based primarily on these considerations. The language of Chinese herbal medicine diagnosis and treatment is distinct from that of modern biomedicine and needs to be under-stood in its own terms. Traditional diagnostic categories such as 'Spleen-Qi deficiency' or 'Liver-Qi stagnation', 'Dampness' or 'Heat in the Blood' are not optional guides, but an integral part of Chinese medicine practice. They de-scribe a clinical reality that, as observed by Charles Buck in the statement quoted above, cannot be reached solely through an understanding of the chemistry. This is why a thorough grounding in the traditional concepts is essential in order to practice Chinese medicine competently. It also explains why it is so difficult to give a satisfactory answer to the question, perfectly legitimate from a biomedical standpoint, 'What's in it and how does it work?' In principle, with sufficient understanding of the pharmacology, this question could perhaps be answered, but that remains a distant prospect.

Safety

A thorough knowledge of the properties of the materia medica as traditionally described is also important in order to practice safely. It was noted in Chapter 3 that the Chinese medicine tradition, from very early times, established clear rules about dosage, about which ingredients may or may not be safely used on a long-term basis, and about which are to be avoided in pregnancy or in paediatric medicine. The special preparation of herbs in order to counteract potency was also developed from very early on. Finally, the construction of a Chinese medicine formula is itself built on the idea of balance, in which the one-sided effects of some ingredients can be counteracted by the addition of others with contrasting qualities.

The use of predictably toxic plant medicines must of course be avoided. However, there are concerns within the herbal medicine community about the use of pharmacological criteria alone in assessing safety. This may lead to an unwarranted focus on chemical constituents seen in isolation, without taking into account the safeguards that are well established within the tradition and that are fundamental features of good Chinese medicine practice. The profession has therefore urged that consideration of safety should recognize the context of herbal practice within which a traditional medicine is used.

The case of *Senecio* and other plant medicines containing pyrrolizidine alkaloids (PAs) provides a good illustration of this point (Box 10.3).

The statutory regulation of herbalists will assist in developing a considered approach to herbal safety. In September 2001, the Medicines Control Agency (MCA, later to become the Medicines and Healthcare Products Regulatory Agency (MHRA)) drew up a list of herbal ingredients about which the agency had 'provisional concerns on public health grounds'. The MCA took the view that regulatory action might be needed either where there was an issue about the inherent toxicity of an ingredient or where the safe use of an ingredient was critically dependent not only on quality control but on factors such as 'competence of the practitioner', 'precise instructions on usage' and 'close monitoring and aftercare' (Medicines Control Agency 2001a). In principle, this could mean that any item that was toxic in its uncooked state, or in a large dose, might be banned on the grounds that there could be no assurance that practitioners would use suitable ingredients or give patients appropriate advice.

The MCA statement was issued at a time when there was no immediate prospect of statutory regulation of herbalists. Statutory regulation is now

> **Box 10.3**   *Senecio* and pyrrolizidine alkaloids
>
> The Register of Chinese Herbal Medicine (RCHM) supported the proposed UK ban on the internal use of *Senecio* species in unlicensed medicines, since the use of these species had been associated with a number of cases of liver damage (Medicines and Healthcare Products Regulatory Agency 2004b). *Senecio* species contain unsaturated PAs, which have been shown to be potentially hepatotoxic. However, the RCHM has stressed that the analysis of isolated ingredients cannot, in most cases, provide sufficient evidence for an evaluation of herbal safety. Evaluation must also take into account the presence of naturally occurring protective buffers within a medicinal plant, the effects of herbal preparation (for example boiling), and the possible protective effects of herbal synergy. In the case of PAs there is evidence that boiling reduces the PA content of a herb by 75–95% (Dharmananda 2001), and that the presence of liquorice root (*Glycyrrhizae uralensis*) in a formula can have a significantly protective effect for the liver (Lin et al 1999). In addition it is important to identify the type of PA involved, because of the wide spectrum of PA toxicity (Register of Chinese Herbal Medicine 2004).

imminent, which will allow the public to identify suitably qualified practitioners and thus provide assurance about the safe use of the materia medica. In addition, as recommended in current proposals for reform of medicines law, certain ingredients that are regarded as especially potent could be restricted to statutorily regulated practitioners (Medicines and Healthcare Products Regulatory Agency 2004b).

Non-plant medicines

The use of non-plant medicines is another issue that has arisen in considering the role of the Chinese medicine tradition (Box 10.4).

RESEARCH

Statutory regulation of the profession and the regulation of herbal products are both primarily concerned with safety. In the longer term though, the strength of herbal medicine, and of CAM therapies as a whole, will depend on their ability to demonstrate efficacy. This raises fundamental questions about appropriate forms of research for herbal medicine and other CAM therapies, each of which is likely to throw up its own particular issues in terms of research design. The challenge is to achieve rigour while ensuring that the design is flexible enough to test what practitioners actually do (Mason et al 2002).

It is widely accepted that the 'gold standard' in research design is reached in double-blind randomized controlled trials (RCTs), and even more so in the meta-analysis of a number of RCTs. These, it is generally agreed, come as close as is possible in the biological sciences to eliminating bias and identifying a

---

Box 10.4   Non-plant medicines

The UK 1968 Medicines Act (section 12) excludes herbal remedies from the need to obtain a medicines licence, but as currently framed this exemption does not apply to non-plant traditional medicines (Medicines Control Agency 2001b). The UK legislation was drawn up at a time when the Chinese tradition, which uses some mineral and animal substances, had almost no presence in the UK, but this position has radically changed over the past 20 years or so. The proposals by the Herbal Medicine Regulatory Working Group on the reform of section 12 (1) included the recommendation that non-plant traditional medicines should be covered in the exemptions provided by the law, so long as the necessary safety and quality standards were met. Following this lead, the MHRA included such an option in its consultation on reform of the law, while stressing particular public health issues associated with non-plant medicines (Medicines and Healthcare Products Regulatory Agency 2004b).

A change in the law relating to non-plant medicines would not affect any restrictions established through the Convention on Trade in Endangered Species. The RCHM, for example, fully supports any restrictions that may be necessary in order to protect endangered species, and its ethical codes strictly forbid the use of any such ingredients by members of the register (Codes of Ethics).

---

causative link between an intervention and an outcome. Analytical observational studies (cohort or case control studies), which can identify important statistical associations, stand somewhere below this in the accepted hierarchy, while case studies occupy the lowliest place, though they are seen as useful in generating hypotheses that can be further investigated by more rigorous methods. Meanwhile, understanding the experience of providing or receiving treatment requires a qualitative approach.

The RCT may indeed be the appropriate design for herbal medicine (though not necessarily for other CAM therapies). However, there are both practical and methodological difficulties that must be taken into account. On the practical side, RCTs are very expensive and time consuming, and it is difficult to gather sufficient patients with comparable conditions to obtain statistically significant results. In addition, difficulties in obtaining funding, combined with the relative lack of research skills among practitioners, tend to perpetuate the weakness of the evidence base when measured in terms of the conventional hierarchy of research values. These difficulties are further compounded by the fact that RCTs are not well suited to assessing chronic degenerative diseases, which require long periods of medical intervention to enable sustained changes to be made. Finally, in their countries of origin, there are ethical difficulties over placebo-controlled trials. Hospitals in China, Japan and Taiwan, where research in Chinese herbal medicine is conducted, may be unwilling to withhold treatments that have become established over hundreds of years. This may help to explain why the controlled trials that commonly appear in Chinese medical journals usually test Chinese herbs not against placebo, but against or in addition to Western drugs.

There are also methodological difficulties, which can in principle be overcome but which require a flexible approach to research design. These difficulties include:

- individualized treatment
- the role of the practitioner
- the treatment of chronic illness.

Individualized treatment

Herbal formulas are tailored to the individual and tend to be modified in the light of patient response to treatment and according to the stage of treatment. It is a regular experience in clinical practice that better results may be gained by modifying a formula in the light of that response. This procedure does not sit well with the normal assumption of standardized treatment in RCTs.

The eczema trials conducted in London in the early 1990s, which were influential in promoting the reputation of Chinese herbal medicine in the treatment of atopic eczema, did not attempt to follow the traditional practice, and instead used a single formula. Chinese medicine principles were to some extent taken into account, since only one broad presentation (non-exudative eczema) was included, and advice was taken from Chinese medicine practitioners about an appropriate formula for this presentation. However, the use of a standardized formula meant that the full potential of the tradition was not tested. The results were impressive, but it is quite possible that with an individualized approach the results would have been even better (Sheehan & Atherton 1992, Sheehan et al 1992).

An Australian team took a different approach in a trial of the treatment of irritable bowel syndrome with Chinese medicine. The team compared a placebo both with a standardized Chinese herbal formula and with treatment that varied according to the individual patient. The conclusion was that both forms of herbal treatment performed significantly better than placebo, and that the benefits of individualized treatment were more sustained than the benefits of standardized treatment (Bensoussan et al 1998). This trial showed one way in which individualized treatment might be incorporated into a rigorous design. A possible limitation was that encapsulated powdered herbs were used, rather than herbal teas. Many practitioners, including the author of this chapter, regard teas as the more effective option. The use of capsules in the Australian study was quite understandable, because treatment with teas poses a serious challenge for blinding, and thus for placebo control. Yet this means that the requirements of gold standard research, seen as the best test of efficacy, may lead to a design that fails to test the full potential of the tradition.

These difficulties are a special case of a well-recognized limitation of RCTs: in order to achieve 'internal' validity, strict criteria of randomization and blinding of patients are applied, but the more rigorously this is done, the more the 'external' validity of the study (its generalizability to the real world of clinical practice) tends to be compromised.

The role of the practitioner

The conventional hierarchy of research design is based on the ideal of assessing the treatment effect while setting aside the influence of the practitioner. However, the role of the practitioner and the relationship between practitioner and patient may be critical in determining outcomes, and may become a key consideration in evaluating the treatment as a whole. If this is not taken into account, an essential element in the treatment process may be missed. One way in which this could be addressed, where more than one practitioner is involved in a trial, is to include stratification by individual practitioner within the randomization process (Mason et al 2002).

The treatment of chronic illness

Herbal medicine and other CAM therapies are often used by people with chronic illnesses that have not responded to conventional treatment. Changes are likely to be slow, and criteria that capture a range of more or less subtle effects need to be established. Such criteria, which may lead towards a qualitative approach, once more may not sit easily with the RCT. Again flexibility is required in establishing outcome measures, and long-term follow-up is needed for results to be meaningful (Mason et al 2002).

THE IMPORTANCE OF OPENNESS AND DIALOGUE

Using Chinese herbal medicine as the focus, the discussion above has stressed the importance of taking into account the specific features of diagnosis and treatment, the traditional understanding of the materia medica, and the problems of research design. All these issues arise from the realities of the clinical encounter in Chinese medicine. They highlight the importance of protecting the knowledge base of the tradition, which is a necessary condition for exploiting its potential to the full.

At the same time, the pursuit of an ideal of pluralism is incompatible with a fortress mentality. Chinese medicine can flourish only if it engages with conventional medicine. This is not a new task, since the tradition has been engaging with Western medicine over a long period. Historically, the Chinese tradition has been characterized by heterogeneity and by a flexible and pragmatic approach to Western medicine (Scheid 2003). This flexibility is apparent in the position of TCM within the present-day Chinese health service. In China, training in Western and Chinese medicine is combined to one degree or another, Chinese medicine practitioners have full legal rights to prescribe a range of pharmaceutical drugs and to conduct biomedical procedures, while Western and Chinese medicine are routinely combined in some form or other.

The heterogeneity and flexibility of the Chinese medicine tradition has been well brought out in the work of Volker Scheid. He has highlighted the plurality of approaches to diagnosis and therapy, arguing also that the definition of medicines as 'systems' or 'paradigms' is not indigenous to the Chinese or other non-Western/non-modern medical traditions. Rather, this conception has been imposed from the outside, in particular by Western observers, in order to describe, classify and control (Box 10.5).

Box 10.5   Heterogeneity in Chinese medicine

Wherever I look in the Chinese medical tradition I cannot find much evidence that physicians ever thought of themselves as practising according to just one particular paradigm. Instead, they were concerned with responding to the vicissitudes of clinical practice in the most flexible way possible. Here is a quote from the *Complete collection of the Four Treasuries* from 1782, a compilation of texts that sought to embody all that was valuable about the Chinese intellectual tradition and thus is as mainstream as it gets:

'Whereas Confucian learning has fixed principles, medical learning does not have fixed methods. [Because the patient's] condition can change in myriad ways, it is impossible to keep to a single tradition.'

Biomedicine itself would never dream of tying itself down to just one paradigm, because that would deny it the flexibility it needs to grow and expand. It does say of course that it is scientific but that is just for appearances. It is scientific when that is suitable and non-scientific when it is not. All available research demonstrates that biomedicine – like all other medicines – is intrinsically diverse, heterogeneous and plural.

(Scheid 2002)

The conclusion drawn by Scheid is not that tradition is unimportant. On the contrary, it is impossible to develop the highest skills in Chinese medicine unless one builds on the classical inheritance. But 'the tradition' presents not a single mode of practice but a multiplicity of styles and testifies to a constant historical development in response to new medical challenges. A corollary is that it is unhelpful to draw tight boundaries between Chinese and Western medicine. The modes of diagnosis and practice are different and these require conditions in which professional autonomy is upheld. But the future of Chinese medicine does not lie in turning backwards or in closing in on itself behind a paradigmatic wall. Rather, the aim is to develop a medical practice that is rooted in tradition yet as open to change as necessary (Scheid 2003).

On this basis, the relationship between the herbal traditions and conventional medicine can be informed by mutual respect while holding true to one's own approach and developing mastery in it. It is in this way that patients will have most to gain.

THE QUESTION OF TRANSLATION

A plural medical world requires communication and understanding between the orthodox and herbal traditions (and, indeed, between different strands within herbal medicine itself). In so far as different medical paradigms are involved, direct translation may not be possible. The use of the term 'paradigm' originates from the work of Thomas Kuhn in the 1960s, which proposed the idea of distinct scientific systems and models (Kuhn 1970). As Simon King points out, however, there are two readings of Kuhn's analysis. On the one hand, he is thought to be saying – a moderate version – that science mostly makes progress, but through debate, where evidence is not always conclusive and non-scientific factors play a part. On the other hand, he is thought to be suggesting an immoderate relativism where changes of paradigm are mostly due to non-empirical factors, and that, once accepted, they radically condition our perception of the world. This second reading suggests that we cannot stand outside paradigms and objectively compare them, which leads to the notion of incommensurability of terms, making translation impossible (King 2002).

The strong version of this argument has a certain attraction to practitioners of Chinese and other traditional forms of medicine struggling to establish a stronger identity within a biomedical world. If we can define a system of medicine to which we belong, and can also opt out of any comparison of its perspective and practice with other paradigms, this might seem to give greater security, even exclusivity, to the knowledge base. However, once we abandon the idea of distinct definable traditions and systems with impermeable boundaries, then the idea of incommensurability weakens. Some form of mutual translation and dialogue between different medical models becomes possible. This has important political implications also: if the concept of paradigm involves a radical separateness, then rational debate becomes impossible, giving Western medicine a free hand to dismiss Chinese medicine as unworthy of serious consideration.

The alternative, as Simon King emphasizes, is a natural evolution alongside Western medicine. The relationship will not be equal, insights from the Chinese tradition will have to be fought for, and some things will be lost as well as won. But this is the creative option for the future (King 2002).

CONCLUSION

The inclusion of Chinese herbal medicine within a framework of statutory regulation is an important and welcome development. Above all, it gives reassurance to patients that practitioners are suitably qualified, up to date and bound by ethical rules. It is also a necessary condition for establishing a closer relationship between conventional and non-conventional healthcare.

At the same time, it is vital that such a statutory framework recognizes the autonomy of different traditions with their corresponding forms of discourse, diagnosis and treatment. Such is the ideal that has been pursued during the many deliberations among herbalists leading up to statutory regulation in the UK. This in itself will not guarantee success, since success comes from the ability to persuade the public, both through everyday clinical practice and through clinical research, that the tradition has something important to offer. However, without such a plural framework it will not be possible to exploit the full potential of the Chinese and other traditions in contemporary healthcare.

References

Acupuncture Regulatory Working Group 2003 The statutory regulation of the acupuncture profession. Prince of Wales's Foundation for Integrated Health, London

Amano T, Hirata A, Namiki M 1996 Effects of Chinese herbal medicine on sperm motility and fluorescence parameters. Archives of Andrology 37(3):219–224

Bensoussan A, Talley N J, Hing M et al 1998 The treatment of irritable bowel syndrome with Chinese herbal medicine: a randomized controlled trial. Journal of the American Medical Association 280(18):1585–1589

Bowling A 2002 Research methods in health. Open University Press, Buckingham

Buck C 2002 In: Protecting the Chinese medicine tradition. RCHM News, October. Register of Chinese Herbal Medicine, London

Chang D et al 1997 The effects of traditional antirheumatic herbal medicines on immune response cells, Journal of Rheumatology. 24(3):436–441

Codes of Ethics 2000 Register of Chinese herbal medicine, London

Department of Health 2004 Regulation of herbal medicine and acupuncture: proposals for statutory regulation. Stationery Office, London

Dharmananda S 2001 Safety issues affecting herbs: pyrrolizidine alkaloids. Online. Available: http://www.itmonline.org/arts/pas.htm

Flower A 2003 A critical evaluation of appropriate research strategies relating to Chinese Herbal Medicine. Unpublished essay.

Government response to the House of Lords Select Committee on Science and Technology's report on Complementary and alternative medicine 2001. Stationery Office, London

Goldsmith M (ed) 1999 2020 vision and NIH heads foresee the future. Journal of the American Medical Association 282(24):2287–2290

Herbal Medicine Regulatory Working Group 2003 Recommendations on the regulation of herbal practitioners in the UK. Prince of Wales's Foundation for Integrated Health, London

House of Lords Select Committee on Science and Technology 2000 Complementary and alternative medicine, 6th report. Stationery Office, London

King S 2002 In: Protecting the Chinese medicine tradition. RCHM News, October. Register of Chinese Herbal Medicine, London

Kuhn T S 1970 The structure of scientific revolutions. University of Chicago Press, Chicago

Lin G, Nnane I P, Cheng T Y 1999 The effects of pre-treatment with glycyrrhizin and glycyrrhetinic acid on the retrorsine-induced hepatotoxicity in rats. Toxicon 37(9):1259–1270

Mason, S, Tovey P, Long A F 2002 Evaluating complementary medicine: methodological challenges of randomised controlled trials. British Medical Journal 325:832–834

Medicines Control Agency 2001a Review of herbal ingredients for use in unlicensed herbal medicinal products. Stationery Office, London

Medicines Control Agency 2001b Traditional ethnic medicines: public health and compliance with medicines law. Stationery Office, London

Medicines and Health Products Regulatory Agency 2004a MLX 296: Proposals to prohibit the sale, supply or importation of unlicensed herbal medicinal products for internal use which contain *Senecio* species. Stationery Office, London

Medicines and Health Products Regulatory Agency 2004b MLX 299: Proposals for the reform of the regulation of unlicensed herbal remedies in the United Kingdom made up to meet the needs of individual patients. Stationery Office, London

Oishi M, Mochizuki Y, Chao E et al 1998 The effectiveness of Traditional Chinese Medicine in Alzheimer disease. Alzheimer Disease and Associated Disorders 12(3):247–250

Rees L, Weil A 2001 Integrated medicine. British Medical Journal 322:119–120

Register of Chinese Herbal Medicine April 2004 Response to MLX 296: Proposals to prohibit the sale, supply or importation of unlicensed herbal medicinal products for internal use which contain *Senecio* species. RCHM, London

Scheid V 2002 In: Protecting the Chinese medicine tradition. RCHM News, October. Register of Chinese Herbal Medicine, London

Scheid V 2003 Chinese medicine in contemporary China. Duke University Press, Durham, NC

Sheehan M, Atherton D 1992 A controlled trial of traditional Chinese medicinal plants in widespread non-exudative atopic eczema. British Journal of Dermatology 126:179–184

Sheehan M P, Rustin M H, Atherton D J et al 1992 Efficacy of traditional Chinese herbal therapy in adult atopic dermatitis Lancet 340:13–17

Suzuki F, Kobayashi M, Komatsu Y et al 1997 Keishi-ka-kei-to, a traditional Chinese herbal medicine, inhibits pulmonary metastasis of B16 melanoma. Anticancer Research 17(2A):873–878

Wright M 2002 In: Protecting the Chinese medicine tradition. RCHM News, October. Register of Chinese Herbal Medicine, London

Yoshida Y, Wang M Q, Liu J N et al 1997 Immunomodulating activity of Chinese medicinal herbs and *Oldenlandia* in particular, International Journal of Immunopharmacology 19(7):59–70

11

Knowledge, skills and competence:
an exploration of the education and professional formation of herbalists

Alison Denham

OVERVIEW

The aim of this chapter is to discuss some issues in the education of prospective herbal practitioners, in the context of the evolution of educational provision over recent years. Each tradition of herbal medicine (Western, Chinese, Ayurvedic and Tibetan) varies in the clinical and diagnostic skills required and the rationale for treatment and prescription of herbal medicine. However, in each case, the aim is for the future practitioner to learn to hold a consultation, develop a therapeutic relationship with the patient and prescribe an individualized herbal prescription. Each tradition has a vitalist element in which bodily function is perceived as dependent on the level and flow of 'energy' (Wood 2000) and an appreciation of this is essential in all traditions.

Educational provision is changing for several reasons. There are the developments in the profession of herbal medicine, which are the subject of this present work. Additionally, there are major changes in higher education for healthcare professionals. Within the profession, there is now greater emphasis on the use of interpersonal skills in the consultation and on enabling more informed choice by the patient. Concurrently there have been significant changes in the education of healthcare professionals in the United Kingdom (Quality Assurance Agency 2001), which also affect education in herbal medicine. Given that, for any programme of study, there are constraints on the provision offered, and resources are finite, this inevitably has created certain tensions. I will also discuss some of the tensions between different aspects of the curriculum and use examples, from experience as a teacher and a practitioner of Western herbal medicine, to show the ongoing creative interplay between education, competence, excellence and reflection.

PROFESSIONAL EDUCATION

Eraut (1994) suggests that there are three distinct characteristics of a profession:

- a specialist knowledge base
- the delivery of a distinctive service
- independence in the exercise of judgement.

A service combines the use of skills and judgement to respond to the individual needs of the client or patient (Barnett 1994). Given that the client or patient has to trust that the service is appropriate, the professional group has an ethical responsibility to both the patient and the public. The aim of the training and education of healthcare practitioners for entry to the profession is to enable the practitioner to practise effectively and safely with an awareness of limits of competence.

There are three main strands to entry-level competence in herbal medicine:

- first, the knowledge and skills required to form a diagnosis and the rationale for treatment and advice
- secondly, the knowledge and skills required to prescribe and dispense safe and effective herbal medicines
- thirdly, the ability to reflect on the patient–practitioner relationship (Herbal Medicine Regulatory Working Group 2003).

The learning appropriate to these three strands is determined differently depending on the particular tradition of herbal medicine. The aim of courses is for the student to learn how to exercise judgement in the development of a treatment plan with the patient. Over a period of only a few years, the exercise of judgement, the delivery of the service and the care given to the patient have changed substantially in response to an increased respect for the rights of the patient to take part in decisions about treatment or care (Greenhalgh 1997). The ethical responsibility of the practitioners to promote the ability of patients to make informed decisions about their healthcare places emphasis on the development of communication skills. The importance of communication skills in the curriculum is likely to increase in the light of the National Professional Standards for Herbal Medicine (2003), which place the establishment and maintenance of effective communications, and respect for the decisions of individuals, at the centre of the consultation.

THE DEVELOPMENT OF PROGRAMMES OF STUDY IN HERBAL MEDICINE

The knowledge base of herbal practice is extensive and representatives of the professional associations affiliated to the European Herbal Practitioners Association (EHPA) began work on a common core curriculum as early as 1992. This became an important strand of the process of working towards a unified profession. The knowledge and skills required for entry-level competence that are required to form a diagnosis and rationale for treatment are specified in the common core curriculum. This document was developed over a period of 8 years by the Education Committee of the EHPA, representing Ayurvedic, Chinese, Western,

Tibetan and Kampo herbal practitioners. It was circulated for consultation in 1999 and the final document agreed in 2000 when all the larger professional associations endorsed the curriculum and agreed to work towards its implementation in programmes of study.

The process of developing a core curriculum (Box 11.1) gave an opportunity for discussion of different aspects of training: clinical skills (traditional and conventional), prescription, the holistic consultation and related subjects such as nutrition. This represented an important stage in the development of the profession as the length and level of existing courses varied. The process required negotiation and compromise between the different traditions and it was valuable to make these issues more explicit.

Box 11.1   The core curriculum

The core curriculum consists of nine sections or elements:

- Human sciences
- Clinical sciences
- Clinical practice
- Nutrition
- Practitioner development and ethics
- Practitioner research
- Plant chemistry and pharmacology
- Pharmacognosy and dispensing.

The final module is the so-called 'eighth element', which is specific to each herbal tradition (Herbal Medicine Regulatory Working Group 2003).

The aim of the curriculum is to provide a framework that both sets minimum levels and also enables course teams to develop an extended curriculum, going beyond the minimum framework. How this happens depends on the tradition and the aims and philosophy of the particular course. For example, there were contested views on the extent of the requirement for an adequate understanding of medical sciences for practitioners of all traditions, although there was agreement that practitioners need to be aware of limits of competence and be able to communicate with patients and other healthcare practitioners. However, in the context of a course in Chinese herbal medicine, an undue emphasis on human sciences would reduce the time spent on traditional methods of diagnosis. It is argued that competence in traditional Chinese diagnostic methods is fundamental to safe practice (Maciocia 2003) and this essential knowledge must not lose its central place in the curriculum. In contrast, courses in Western herbal medicine would be expected, within the philosophy of the particular course, to give substantially more time to human sciences as students are expected to be able to relate the actions of herbs to the underlying physiology.

An important part of the process of agreeing the core curriculum was for each tradition to agree the 'eighth element', a tradition-specific element that sets out the philosophy, materia medica and distinctive characteristics particular to that tradition (Herbal Medicine Regulatory Working Group 2003). Thus the eighth element is a major section in the curriculum for each tradition. The module goes far beyond the prescribing of herbs as it encompasses the rationale underlying the therapeutic strategy. Each herbal tradition is based on the transmission of clinical experience through oral teaching, through textbooks written by practitioners and through journal articles written by practitioners. It is the skilful use of such material that enables the practitioner to design a prescription for the individual patient (Box 11.2). Within all traditions, it is usual for prescribing methods to vary substantially between practitioners and to depend, not just on the disease, but also on the patient's symptoms and constitution.

Box 11.2   Competence in prescribing: the underpinning knowledge base

To explain the breadth of knowledge required for competent prescribing, I will discuss the evidence base for the Western tradition of herbal medicine, which encompasses European, North American and some tropical medicinal plants. Practitioners are required to understand conventional disease processes, the therapeutic strategy and prescription but also require an understanding of the underlying energetic and tissue state in the light of earlier herbal theories such as Physiomedicalism (Cook 1985), which drew from humoral theories of medicine (Tobyn 1997). Prescribing in Western herbal medicine continues to be influenced by Greco-Roman practice (Arber 1995) and texts that set down oral knowledge (Bryce 1988, Culpeper 1995). There is also increasing evidence for prescribing based on scientific and clinical research (Blumenthal 2000, Rotblatt & Irwin 2002), and an understanding of herbal pharmacology underpins the safe prescribing of medicinal plants (Bruneton 1999, Mills & Bone 2000). In addition, an understanding of botanical identification of plant material (Bradley 1993) is required to understand the significance of quality assurance in sourcing medicinal plants. Students must also be aware of safety issues and the monitoring of the safety of herbal medicines (Shaw et al 1997) and of potential drug–herb interactions (Izzo & Ernst 2001), knowledge of which has increased over recent years.

In addition to learning how to prescribe, students are required to be able to form a care plan and the therapeutic strategy will also include advice on diet, lifestyle (Eldin & Dunford 1999) and other more spiritual aspects of holistic healthcare. As part of a course team, I have had extensive discussions about the appropriate knowledge and skills required by the practitioner after graduation. Herbal practitioners treat an enormous range of conditions, both acute and chronic, which could be classified into three categories to clarify teaching and learning objectives:

● first, common conditions (such as eczema or premenstrual tension), which require the practitioner to advise on lifestyle as well as prescribe for the individual

- secondly, relatively common but serious conditions (such as rheumatoid arthritis or endometriosis), which require the practitioner to understand both conventional and complementary opinions on care
- thirdly, rare or unusual conditions where the patient may consult the herbal practitioner because other proposed treatment options are limited.

No curriculum can cover everything but students of herbal medicine can be expected to form a working diagnosis for common and more serious conditions, and to be aware of the need to review reference material in rare or unusual conditions. In all three categories, it is essential that students keep abreast of published research in prescribing, conventional and complementary approaches to healthcare, and dietary and lifestyle advice (Denham 1998). The ability to modify practice in the light of new research, professional and academic debate is important; and herbal practitioners need to continue to update their skills, and to use online sources of evidence, as one may spend a considerable time discussing the evidence base for diagnosis and treatment.

The significance of the emphasis on enabling patient choice has increased since the Department of Health's (1998) recommendations to put the interests of patients explicitly at the centre of healthcare. In that context, the future practitioner has also to learn to be impartial, to recognize limits of competence (General Medical Council 2001) and not to be afraid to advise the patient to seek conventional treatment or treatment by another complementary practitioner. Emphasis on the importance of informed choice, and thus informed consent, has increased since the publication of the Bristol Royal Infirmary Inquiry (2001). One recommendation was the formation of an overarching body with a mandate to make professional self-regulation more consistent and more accountable to the patient, the public and government (Council for the Regulation of Healthcare Professionals 2001). There is an opinion among herbalists that the development of statutory regulation and public accountability could diminish the quality of care in complementary medicine if it were to result in less individualized patient care. In my experience, debate between patient and practitioner in discussion of the care plan is an enriching process.

Allowing students to develop into practitioners who are able to reflect on their own practice is a first step towards encouraging practitioners to develop and retain a sensitive relationship with patients. Although the concept of the reflective practitioner is not new (Schon 1987), the development of reflection is now increasingly explicit within the curriculum. In common with other healthcare professions, training in herbal medicine has been changing over the last 20 years. It is no longer possible merely to acquire knowledge and skills 'in vacuo', divorced from an understanding of the patient/practitioner relationship (Katz 2000). Courses have to aim to produce practitioners who are able to communicate with patients, to respect the autonomy of patients and to establish a relationship of trust with the patient (Mitchell & Cormack 1998). The competencies required for herbal practitioners (Herbal Medicine Regulatory Working Group 2003, p. 44) therefore begin with a list of nine professional values and behaviours. One can see this emphasis on values throughout training in the healthcare professions. For example, the Quality Assurance Agency subject benchmark for degrees in medicine states that graduates must 'adopt an empathic and holistic approach to patients and the problems they present' (Quality Assurance Agency 2002, p. 6).

It is also a requirement that graduates demonstrate the ability to apply their knowledge in the professional situation (Cowan 1998). For example, curriculum standards for the proposed approval process for courses leading to registration by the Health Professions Council state 'The delivery of the programme assists autonomous and reflective thinking and evidence based practice' (Health Professions Council 2004, p. 8).

In the EHPA core curriculum, clinical training, which requires direct contact with patients in the clinical setting, is integrated into courses from the first or second year. There is an explicit effort to link theory and practice in the EHPA core curriculum, which integrates academic and technical learning within the context of clinical practice. This can allow the student to progress through stages of learning (Cowan 1998) as it provides concrete experience of supervised practice. Cowan (1998) argues that the provision of real-life examples enables the future professional to learn how to reflect on practice. The assessment structure needs to link theory with practice and requires learners to demonstrate both theoretical and practical knowledge leading to analysis, synthesis and the creative application of theory and practice (Herbal Medicine Regulatory Working Group 2003). In common with other healthcare professions (Watson et al 2002), assessment of clinical competence in herbal practice is evolving in the light of current debate. Such debate is essential in the evolution of the education of new entrants to the herbal profession. Biggs (1999) argues that the integration of theoretical and practical learning based on explicit discussion and determination of objectives leads to an alignment of teaching and learning activities, curriculum objectives and assessment. This in turn promotes improved learning and thus the eventual ability of the graduate to develop into an effective practitioner.

APPROVAL OF COURSES IN HERBAL MEDICINE

The accreditation or approval of courses leading to professional qualifications in healthcare is the mechanism whereby the profession sets the standards for entry to the professional register. The public is thus enabled to make an informed choice of qualified practitioner from the register, which is published and administered by a statutory body or a voluntary professional association. Therefore, accreditation of courses depends on explicit guidelines not just for educational standards, knowledge and skills but also for the attitudes and personal attributes required of a qualified practitioner. The goal of accreditation is to ensure that newly qualified practitioners are competent to practice, with the proviso that course provision at any college will vary in ethos, content and teaching and learning strategy.

Historically, course accreditation procedures developed from the inspection of courses by professional associations. The development of accreditation boards in herbal medicine ensured a separation of responsibilities between the councils of the respective professional associations and those involved in running schools or in the accreditation of courses. Such a development is not widespread throughout complementary medicine. However, accreditation is a fundamental stage in voluntary professional self-regulation, leading to transparency in the setting and enforcement of standards of education and training (Champion 2002).

From their inception, accreditation boards in herbal medicine have had lay chairs and included educationalists from outside the profession. It is perhaps fortunate that accreditation of courses in herbal medicine did not develop until the 1990s with the result that policies have, from the outset, encouraged variety in ethos and content. This partly reflected the major changes being introduced in training in conventional healthcare as demonstrated by the review (General Medical Council 2000) by medical schools of their curriculum, development of skills and attitudes, communication skills and learning systems in response to the original proposals in 'Tomorrow's doctors'. The first move towards accreditation of training courses in herbal medicine occurred in 1994 when the National Institute of Medical Herbalists (NIMH) began to prepare the necessary documentation and to establish a constitution for an accreditation board. The 10-member board was set up in 1996 with the aim of promoting standards of training that ensure the good practice of herbal medicine and, in dialogue with training institutions, both recognize and develop good quality theoretical and practical education (National Institute of Medical Herbalists 2000).

Once progress had been made on the EHPA core curriculum, it was recognized that, as part of its work towards a unified profession, the EHPA should form an accreditation board able to accredit courses from any tradition within a framework which 'recognises and values the diverse ethnic and cultural philosophies of herbal medicine' (Herbal Medicine Regulatory Working Group 2003, p. 41). The principals of the schools that provided graduates were in agreement and, in early 1998, the member professional associations agreed to a common accreditation process. The EHPA Accreditation Board was founded in 2000, with the support of the Prince of Wales's Foundation for Integrated Health in the appointment of a lay Chair, which has proved invaluable in its development. The accreditation process relies on documentary reviews of:

- course content
- quality assurance procedures

- finance
- management
- resources
- the policies of the school.

This is combined with visits to training establishments to meet with students and staff. If appropriate, the EHPA Accreditation Board relates professional accreditation to the process of academic validation of courses by universities and undertakes joint events where possible. Validation refers to the internal mechanisms in place within universities to approve new courses. Many existing courses are within well-established schools or universities and the prior achievement of external or internal validation shows that course developers have already made explicit decisions about course philosophy, content and academic provision. This close relationship between the accreditation and the validation approach is in line with the consultation on determining criteria and procedures for the approval (equivalent to accreditation) of courses undertaken by the Health Professions Council (2004). Cooperative accreditation and validation is also advocated by the Quality Assurance Agency for Higher Education (2004) in the 'Partnership Quality Assurance Framework for Healthcare Education in England: a consultation', which proposes common standards and methods of quality assurance of healthcare education through both approval processes and ongoing quality monitoring and enhancement.

The aim of the EHPA Board is to ensure common standards, but it also has a responsibility to the different traditions within herbal medicine to build a framework that both recognizes and values diverse ethnic and cultural philosophies (Herbal Medicine Regulatory Working Group 2003). In addition, the practitioners who developed the EHPA core curriculum were anxious to protect the independent schools, which have kept the tradition of herbal medicine alive in the United Kingdom. An implication of this is the requirement for course provision to support quality student learning without making the associated financial costs too high for an independent school, which is not part of the publicly funded higher education sector in the UK. In particular, it is envisaged that full-time courses, part-time courses and distance-learning courses will be accredited to allow for flexibility in patterns of delivery, and to support institutional autonomy and student choice.

As a member professional association of the EHPA, the NIMH agreed to the formation of a unified accreditation process, adopted the EHPA core curriculum as its minimum standard and undertook to reassess the role of the NIMH Accreditation Board. In the event, there proved to be unanticipated difficulties in managing the changes in working practice and in the formation of the constitution of the EHPA Accreditation Board. At the time of writing, discussion is continuing between the two boards to seek agreement on procedures to transfer accreditation of courses to the EHPA Accreditation Board. However, in 2004, it was agreed that NIMH would recognize the graduates of courses accredited by the EHPA for entry on to the NIMH register. As President of NIMH for part of the time that this process was under discussion, my observation is that any change has different implications for different parties. The work and discussion needed to unravel the required changes in procedures and administration can be complex. It is helpful to the process of creating a unified herbal profession that some of these problems are being addressed now rather than after the formation of a statutory register.

CURRENT COURSE PROVISION IN WESTERN HERBAL MEDICINE

Having reviewed the development of the curriculum and the accreditation of courses for prospective herbal practitioners, I will now discuss some of the issues arising in course provision by examining the development of courses in Western herbal medicine. Entrance to the NIMH has been by examination since 1908. Until 1982, it accepted only applicants who had completed the NIMH training course. After 1982, the training course, which at this time was a 4-year distance-learning course, was taken over by an independent school, the College of Phytotherapy. The College gained external validation for a full-time course in 1995 and for a new distance-learning course in 1997. There are now 120 students registered on their programmes and it is one of two private schools that are externally validated by universities. The other is the Scottish School of Herbal Medicine, which was formed in 1992 with the intention of providing an education based on holistic principles. That course is delivered part time over 4 years. Part-time and distance-learning courses can be particularly suitable for students who already hold other qualifications. Such delivery methods provide a means to widen access to training in herbal medicine for those institutions that may struggle to offer the more traditional, in higher education terms, 3-year full-time routes.

Private schools do not have the resource base of universities. One school, the Self-Heal School, took the decision that it was not appropriate to continue to enrol students, as it was not sure that it would achieve the new standards set by the accreditation process. The Self-Heal School was established in 1994 to develop further the training courses that had been offered since 1982 by the British branch of Dr Christopher's American School of Natural Healing. It trained some 65 graduates in its 9-year life and gave particular emphasis to the associated use of naturopathic methods such as dietary regimens, exercise and hydrotherapy. However, the managing committee of the school, being fully committed to the development of high standards in education and training, felt that operating as an independent school was no longer the best way to fulfil their mission.

There are now seven full-time degree-level courses offered by universities in the UK and this has enhanced the quality and research base of education in herbal medicine. The provision of courses in herbal medicine within higher education has a number of exciting implications. These include the opportunity:

- to increase research into the practice of herbal medicine
- to promote self-reflection and analysis of the role of the practitioner in complementary medicine
- to reinvestigate traditional Western herbal medicines.

However, the move into higher education since 1994 of Western herbal medicine training courses has introduced further academic and educational requirements. To achieve an honours degree (Quality Assurance Agency 2001), the student must:

- evaluate the evidence base
- evaluate the associated research methods
- demonstrate critical thinking in reaching sound judgements
- demonstrate progression over the course
- undertake a dissertation.

The modular provision of courses, and assessment of learning outcomes, allows for a clear progression in skills, knowledge and in the ability to integrate analysis and application. For course teams, it is a challenge to provide a curriculum within a 3-year, 18-module course that combines adequate knowledge, skills, personal development and academic learning. In addition, the move into higher education is increasing the number of school leavers who enter the profession and the range of academic background of applicants. The government and university policy of widening participation (Admissions to Higher Education Review 2003, Higher Education Funding Council for England 2004) means that course teams have a responsibility to ensure both that applications are treated equally and that students are supported so that they progress to a degree (Floud 2002). For course teams, this means that a balance has to be found between this policy and the requirement to produce a competent and safe practitioner (Ilott & Murphy 1999). In addition, there is an added responsibility to ensure that everything possible is done to help students to cope with the demands of the varied curriculum (Doel et al 2002, Gamache 2002). In the past, many students were making a career change and had already been educated to degree or diploma level before entering courses in herbal medicine. This still remains common, so that some classes include students with widely differing academic backgrounds from access courses to students with postgraduate qualifications.

The first degree in herbal medicine provided within higher education was a 4-year course. It was later revalidated as a 3-year extended semester course, which is now the usual length. Honours degrees in Scotland last for 4 years, which provides a longer period for the student to develop and mature. In practice, this means that course teams have to tread a middle path between ensuring that an adequate knowledge base is acquired and developing the communication skills and understanding of the patient–practitioner relationship that is necessary to be able to apply the knowledge in the clinical context (Richardson 2001). In addition, in common with other practical degree courses, the inclusion of skill-based learning in the form of clinical training makes resourcing the programme difficult for universities, as the overall core grants are determined by the Higher Education Funding Council for England. Within a finite provision of teaching time, there is an inevitable tension between knowledge, skills and reflection within the curriculum. This is not unique to complementary medicine and occurs in training for many professional qualifications. Pickering (2000) suggests that the facilitation of reflection is essential to enable practitioners to continue to reflect and thus embrace change and innovation through their professional life. Cowan (1998) argues that the provision of opportunities for students to reflect on their learning linked with assessment that requires the student to demonstrate their reflection will enable graduates to leave university with both knowledge and the means to apply that knowledge as a professional practitioner.

Barnett (1994) argues that an emphasis on competence, skills and measurable learning outcomes threatens the development of students' understanding, which, he suggests, should be at the heart of higher education. He describes understanding as a state of consciousness, 'an inner grasp' (Barnett 1994, p. 99), which thus cannot be measured. Understanding then requires not only knowledge and critical thinking but to be 'sensitive to hidden significances, delicate shifts of emphasis and nuances of expression' (Elliott 1975, cited in Barnett 1994). The inclusion of a dissertation may go some way towards initiating the journey to understanding, particularly if it embraces current debate over the more complex issues in complementary medicine such as appropriate research methods (Lewith et al 2002) or subtle interactions in the healing relationship (Peters 2001).

The degree course is only the first step in professional formation and it provides a more secure foundation if that is explicitly recognized. My experience in planning the content of teaching sessions in therapeutics is that it has been helpful to recall that training is leading to entry-level competence. This awareness has enabled the setting of clearer and more achievable learning outcomes. It is possible to maintain a formal structure yet also inculcate the will to continue to question (Biggs 1999), and thus embark on what is often now called the process of lifelong learning.

CONTINUING PROFESSIONAL DEVELOPMENT

Continuing professional development (CPD) has been mandatory within most professional associations in herbal medicine for some years now and the current emergence of postgraduate education in complementary medicine can only promote this process.

As the report of the Herbal Medicine Regulatory Working Group (2003) states, it is expected that all healthcare practitioners will be covered by mandatory continuing professional development, which will enable practitioners both to maintain and to increase skills, knowledge and professional activity. The CPD programme for practitioners of herbal medicine (Herbal Medicine Regulatory Working Group 2003 Annexe 5) is designed to be flexible and inclusive and to include a wide range of appropriate learning. The provision of participatory continuing professional development by professional associations poses some challenges. Most herbal practitioners are self-employed, many live in rural areas, and many (both women and men) have caring responsibilities, making participation in formal programmes of CPD problematic. However, it is a challenge that has to be met. CPD programmes that provide lifelong learning for all clinicians and healthcare workers are one of the five elements in the Department of Health policy on clinical governance (Department of Health 1998). The focus of this policy is quality of care within the National Health Service, but the principles underlying clinical governance are relevant throughout healthcare (Van Zwanenburgh & Harrison 2000) and statutory registers are moving towards the linkage of mandatory CPD with professional revalidation (General Medical Council 2004).

CONCLUSION

The tensions between excellence and the core knowledge and competence required for safe practice will continue to shape the provision of education for herbal practitioners. Excellence can be expressed as the development of the traditional art of herbal medicine by reflective, holistic practitioners. Competence for safe practice incorporates contemporary notions of safety, efficacy and patient-centredness within NHS good practice, as well as traditional understanding of these issues. These tensions in professional education could provide the challenge needed to move towards a form of provision that responds to those current theories of learning that argue that students learn through the undertaking of activities (Biggs 1999).

Most courses in higher education can be evaluated in the light of subject benchmark statements, which provide a statement of programme requirements (Quality Assurance Agency 2002) and in the light of professional standards of proficiency such as those published by the Health Professions Council (2003). An attempt has been made to produce subject benchmark statements in complementary medicine but this has not yet proved possible, probably because too broad a range of therapies was included. However, the National Professional Standards for Herbal Medicine (2003) have been agreed and could provide the groundwork for benchmarking in herbal medicine. These standards have built on the EHPA core curriculum in giving emphasis to the development of the holistic practitioner as a person with the ability to reflect on, and respond to, the needs of the wider society and communicate with the patient on a wide range of health-related issues. This reflects the growing awareness of the requirement to inculcate in students the values and attitudes that will promote lifelong learning. The balance between knowledge, skills and ethos is not fixed, and we need to educate practitioners who are able to adapt to changing circumstances within healthcare. The relative recency of the evolution of validated and accredited courses in herbal medicine provides an opportunity to develop courses according to current thinking in learning and teaching and to promote high-quality patient care through herbal medicine.

References

Admissions to Higher Education Review 2003 Terms of reference. Online. Available: www.admissions-review.org.uk 7 April 2004

Arber A 1995 Herbals: their origin and evolution. Cambridge University Press, Cambridge

Barnett R 1994 The limits of competence. Open University Press, Buckingham

Biggs J 1999 Teaching for quality learning at university. Open University Press, Buckingham

Blumenthal M (ed) 2000 Herbal medicine: expanded Commission E monographs. Integrative Medicine Communications, Massachusetts

Bradley P (ed) 1993 British herbal compendium. British Herbal Medicine Association, London

Bristol Royal Infirmary Inquiry 2001 Learning from Bristol: the report of the public inquiry into children's heart surgery at the Bristol Royal Infirmary 1984–1995. Command paper: CM 5207. Online. Available: www.bristol-inquiry.org.uk 12 May 2004

Bruneton J 1999 Pharmacognosy, phytochemistry, medicinal plants. Lavoisier Publishing, Paris

Bryce D (ed) 1988 The herbal remedies of the physicians of Myddfai. Llanerch, Dyfed

Champion R 2002 Good practice in accreditation. The Prince of Wales's Foundation for Integrated Health complementary therapies workshop on accreditation 15 February 2002. Online. Available: http://www.fihealth.org.uk/fs_what_we_do.html 12 May 2004

Cook W 1869, reprinted 1985 The physio-medical dispensatory. Eclectic Medical Publications, Oregon

Council for the Regulation of Healthcare Professionals 2001 Functions. Online. Available: www.crhp.org.uk 12 May 2004

Cowan J 1998 On becoming an innovative university teacher. Open University Press, Buckingham

Culpeper N 1641 (edition published 1995) Culpeper's complete herbal. Wordsworth Editions, Hertfordshire

Denham A 1998 Clinical audit report: introducing patient care plans based on a clinical question. European Journal of Herbal Medicine 4(2):25–31

Department of Health 1998 A first class service: quality in the new NHS. Stationery Office, London.

Doel M, Sawdon C, Morrison D 2002 Learning, practice and assessment: signposting the portfolio. Jessica Kingsley, London.

Eldin S, Dunford A 1999 Herbal medicine in primary care. Butterworth-Heinemann, Oxford

Eraut M 1994 Developing professional knowledge and competence. Falmer, London

Floud R 2002 Policy implications of student non-completion: government, funding councils and universities. In: Peelo M, Wareham T (eds) Failing students in higher education. Open University Press, Buckingham, p 56–72

Gamache P 2002 University students as creators of personal knowledge; an alternative epistemological view. Teaching in Higher Education 7(3):277–294

General Medical Council 2000 Changing times, changing culture: 5-year review of the work of the General Medical Council. General Medical Council, London

General Medical Council 2001 Good medical practice. Online. Available: www.gmc-uk.org/standards/default.htm 13 May 2004

General Medical Council 2004 Continuing professional development. Online. Available: www.gmc-uk.org New CPD guidance 13 May 2004

Greenhalgh T 1997 How to read a paper. BMJ Publishing Group, London

Health Professions Council 2003 Standards of proficiency. Online. Available:
www.hpc-uk.org/registrants/sop.htm 13 May 2004

Health Professions Council 2004 Standards of education and training and
the approvals process: a consultation paper. Online. Available:
www.hpc-uk.org.uk/consultation/set_approvals 12 April 2004

Herbal Medicine Regulatory Working Group 2003 Recommendations on the
regulation of herbal practitioners. Prince of Wales's Foundation for Integrated
Health, London

Higher Education Funding Council for England 2004 Widening participation. Online.
Available: www.hefce.ac.uk/widen 7 April 04

Ilott I, Murphy R 1999 Success and failure in professional education: assessing the
evidence. Whurr Publications, London

Izzo A, Ernst E 2001 Interactions between herbal medicines and prescribed drugs.
Drugs 61(15):2163–2175

Katz T 2000 University education for developing professional practice In: Bourner T,
Katz T, Watson D (eds) New directions in professional higher education. Open
University Press, Buckingham, p 19–32

Lewith G, Jonas W, Walach H (eds) 2002 Clinical research in complementary therapies.
Churchill Livingstone, London

Maciocia G 2003 Diagnosis in Chinese medicine. Elsevier, London

Mills S, Bone K 2000 Principles and practice of phytotherapy. Churchill Livingstone,
London

Mitchell A, Cormack M 1998 The therapeutic relationship in complementary medicine.
Churchill Livingstone, Edinburgh

National Institute of Medical Herbalists 2000 Accreditation board constitution.
National Institute of Medical Herbalists, Exeter

National Professional Standards for Herbal Medicine 2003. Online. Available:
www.skillsforhealth.org.uk/standards_database/index 12 April 2004

Peters D (ed) 2001 Understanding the placebo effect in complementary medicine.
Churchill Livingstone, London

Pickering A 2000 Independent reflection in teacher education. In: Bourner T, Katz T,
Watson D (eds) New directions in professional higher education. Open University
Press, Buckingham, p 74–82

Quality Assurance Agency for Higher Education 2001 National qualification
framework. Online. Available: www.qaa.ac.uk/crntwork/nqf/ewni2001.htm
13 April 2004

Quality Assurance Agency for Higher Education 2002 Subject benchmark statements.
Online. Available: www.qaa.ac.uk/crntwork/benchmark/phase2/medicine 13 April
2004

Quality Assurance Agency for Higher Education 2004 Partnership quality assurance
framework for healthcare in England: a consultation. Online. Available:
www.qaa.ac.uk/health/consultation/consultation/set_approvals.htm 7 April 2004

Richardson J 2001 Intersubjectivity and the therapeutic relationship. In: Peters D (ed)
Understanding the placebo effect in complementary medicine. Churchill
Livingstone, London, p 13–146

Rotblatt M, Irwin Z 2002 Evidence based herbal medicine. Hanley & Belfus, Philadelphia

Schon D 1987 Educating the reflective practitioner. Jossey-Bass, San Francisco

Shaw D Leon C, Kolev S et al 1997 Traditional remedies and food supplements. Drug
Safety 17(5):324–356

Tobyn, G 1997 Culpeper's medicine. Element Books, Shaftesbury

Van Zwanenburgh T, Harrison J 2000 Clinical governance in primary care. Radcliffe Medical Press, Oxford

Watson R, Stimpson A, Topping A et al 2002 Clinical competence assessment in nursing: a systematic review of the literature. Journal of Advanced Nursing 39(5):421–431

Wood M 2000 Vitalism: the history of herbalism, homeopathy and flower essences. North Atlantic Books, Berkeley

12

Knowledge and myths of knowledge in the 'science' of herbal medicine

Peter Conway

OVERVIEW

The process of exploring regulatory options for herbal practitioners has, as one might expect, stimulated a degree of reflection on core issues pertaining to the profession, its identity and meanings. Discussions on fundamental topics have taken place within the European Herbal Practitioners Association (EHPA), the Herbal Medicine Regulatory Working Group (HMRWG) and the herbal professional associations. Epistemological considerations have frequently come to the fore, revolving around debates over what we think we know about herbal medicine and how we think that we know it.

This has especially been the case because the EHPA has provided the first forum in which the various traditions of herbal medicine have been drawn together to focus solely on the development of the profession as a whole. However, such debate has rarely been extensive and is poorly documented in formal sources, although discussion touching on the wide variety of subjects concerning knowledge in herbal medicine has taken place additionally in conferences, internal newsletters and email groups. The aim of this chapter is to review the current epistemological issues in herbal medicine with a primary emphasis on Western herbal medicine, since this is the author's own area of expertise. Since some of the areas of debate below are not recorded in any formal literature, and because of the nature of the issues concerned, the author presents a personal view drawing on his close involvement with the regulatory process. It is hoped and intended that readers will engage critically with many of the statements and opinions voiced here.

WHOSE KNOWLEDGE?

It is sometimes galling for herbal practitioners to hear herbal medicine classified as a form of 'alternative' or 'complementary' therapy; that is to say as a form of 'non-conventional' medicine. If one looks at medicine as a whole, from both an historical and a contemporary global perspective, then a case can be made for considering herbal medicine as the most conventional of all forms of medicine. The estimation in a Bulletin of the World Health Organization (Farnsworth et al 1985) that 80% of the world's population relies on plant-derived medicines for primary healthcare needs has frequently been cited in the herbal literature. A more recent WHO document (World Health Organization 2003) has calculated that up to 80% of the population in Africa uses traditional medicines for primary healthcare and that, in China, herbal medicines account for 30–50% of total medicines consumption. It goes on to state that the annual global expenditure on herbal medicines is over US$60 billion and that in the UK and North America over 50% of the population has used some form of complementary and alternative medicine (CAM) at least once.

Practitioner consultations and the demand for herbal medicines

Barnes (2000) attempted to assess how demand for herbal medicines might translate into demand for consultations with herbal practitioners in the UK. She cited a Consumer's Association study which revealed that, of 20 000 individuals surveyed in 1995, 31% had consulted a complementary therapist at some time, and of these 6% had consulted a herbal practitioner in the last 12 months. She adds that:

"It is not easy to obtain a clear picture of the use of medical herbalists from these figures; however, if it is assumed that all other individuals surveyed had not consulted a medical herbalist in the previous 12 months, then the 163 individuals who had done so represent less than 1 per cent of the total sample ..."

(Barnes 2000)

A later study looking at the use of herbal medicines in England showed that, whereas 20% of the sample (of 5000 adults) had bought an over-the-counter (OTC) herbal medicine in the last year, only 1% had consulted a herbal practitioner (Thomas et al 2001).

There is a clear discrepancy between the demand for herbal medicines and the demand for consultations with herbal practitioners. The vast majority of herbal medicines consumed in the UK are taken as OTC medicines rather than as medicines prescribed by herbal practitioners. This is perhaps unsurprising given the current size of the profession in the UK. Calculating from figures given for numbers of practitioners listed in professional herbal medicine association registers in the HMRWG Report (Herbal Medicine Regulatory Working Group 2003), the size of the voluntarily regulated herbal profession in the UK (across all traditions) was 1610 practitioners in 2003. The figure may be somewhat lower, however, since some practitioners belong to more than one register. Of the given number, 809 could be placed in the category of Western herbal medicine, 724 as Chinese medicine and 77 as Ayurvedic medicine practitioners. There are no figures for Tibetan medicine or Kampo (traditional Japanese medicine), or other traditions of herbal medicine, which do not exist as substantial entities in the UK at the present time.

In conventional medicine, the same general situation occurs in that medicines may be accessed via consultations with doctors or OTC in pharmacies.

However, there is far less disparity between the two sources in this case and there is a good degree of understanding on the part of the public about which way of obtaining conventional medicines is most appropriate for them, depending on their needs. Although there is little research in this area, it is the author's experience that the public perception of herbal practitioners – who they are and what they do – is very low. Herbalism is commonly mistaken for homeopathy and the public may think of herbalists (if they think of them at all) as herbal shopkeepers or herbal pharmacists (perhaps even as apothecaries).

There is an inherent tension here since herbal practitioners will contend that they are the holders of the true knowledge of herbal medicine, but consumers of herbal medicine may only rarely have contact with them and even be unaware of their existence as a body of professionals. There is a conflict between the idea of herbal medicine as a globally conventional practice of medicine and the actuality of the locally (UK) marginal nature of herbal practitioners. In the absence of practitioners properly inhabiting the territory that they feel to be theirs, the voices of those from outside the profession may assume a higher level of visibility and credibility. The central role of the practitioner will thus often go unrecognized; this can lead to a sense of frustration and disconnection for practitioners, leading to demoralization, a sense of vulnerability and sometimes a resulting knee-jerk protectionism.

Most of the conventionally recognized guides to the use of herbal medicines are written by pharmacists (e.g. Fetrow & Avila 2001, Newall et al 1996). Although this might raise the ire of herbal practitioners (including the author, Conway 2001), because of the lack of a practitioner perspective in such texts, the situation is perhaps understandable given the status of herbal medicine in the UK as a largely OTC phenomenon.

The viability of the proposition that herbal practitioners are the leading experts on herbal medicine and the holders of the true knowledge of herbal medicine is therefore questionable, given that the majority of herbal medicine transactions taking place in the UK are independent of herbal practitioners. It may be more appropriate to contend that herbal practitioners, each according to their own tradition and persuasion, are the holders of a particular strand of knowledge about herbal medicine. Certainly it is not only herbalists who use plants as medicines, they are also used in:

- aromatherapy (volatile or essential oils)
- homeopathy and flower essences
- nutritional medicine
- naturopathy
- and, of course, conventional medicine.

The fact that they are not used in the same ways or within the same terms of reference does not alter the fact that all of the above practices could be considered to some extent to be types of 'herbal medicine'. Herbal medicine might therefore be considered a highly (one might even say wildly) pluralistic entity, when viewed in the broadest sense. Certainly the above modalities, (alongside other groups with an interest in herbal medicines such as manufacturers, suppliers and retailers), have been acknowledged as stakeholders in herbal medicine and involved in the regulatory consultation process.

Differences between traditions

Within the more narrowly defined sphere of herbal medicine as it is normally considered, there are marked points of departure between traditions as well as significant areas of commonality. The two main practices of herbal medicine in the UK (Chinese herbal medicine and what we might, by comparison, call Western herbal medicine) differ fundamentally on the key point of what is meant by the term 'herbal medicine'. In Western herbal medicine, this term is generally restricted to the use of medicinal plants. In Chinese medicine, it usually additionally incorporates other medicinal substances such as minerals and animal parts. Not only does this difference exist, but also many Western practitioners are profoundly opposed to the use of animals as medicinal substances (see Chapter 8). This major difference on a fundamental issue highlights the inappropriateness of speaking of a single body of definitive herbal knowledge. The nature of knowledge can change, depending on one's approach and perspective. It is therefore more appropriate to talk about the professions, in the plural, of herbal medicine than to view herbal medicine as a single cohesive body.

The practice of herbal medicine overall is in the position of being one of the oldest occupations in this country, and having the status of an emerging profession in the UK. There is a difference here, however, between Western herbal medicine and other herbal traditions such as Chinese herbal medicine and Indian Ayurvedic medicine. The last two cases have clearly differing origins and principles when compared with Western conventional scientific medicine, whereas that cannot be said for Western herbal medicine. In the latter case, the origins and, to some extent the principles and practice, of the two are more entangled. Additionally, the Chinese and Ayurvedic traditions can demonstrate ancient roots and a coherent history of practice. The Western herbal tradition is less easily discerned, being more tied up with that of Western conventional medicine. The following section considers the relationship between Western herbal medicine and Western conventional medicine, and its relationship with Western scientific thinking.

Comparing knowledge: Western herbal medicine and Western conventional medicine

In the early 1900s, the materia medica of conventional medicine comprised largely plant drugs (see, for instance, Barclay 1909) and this situation continued until as late as the 1940s (General Medical Council 1948, Hindes 1940). Botany was still taught in some British medical schools until the 1950s, and pharmacognosy continues to be studied as a branch of pharmacy. Even today:

"25% of modern prescription drugs contain at least one compound now or once derived or patterned after compounds derived from higher plants."

(Duke 1993)

To this extent, we can say that conventional medicine continues to utilize plants as healing resources. Conventional Western medicine and Western herbal medicine essentially shared the same history until recent times (Barker 2001). Hippocrates (or rather proponents of the Hippocratic school), Dioscorides, Galen and Avicenna were significant in the development of both. Although herbal practitioners can justifiably claim these figures as great 'herbalists' they were in fact physicians, using a variety of substances (not just plants) and strategies to care for their patients.

THE MYTH OF PURE HERBAL MEDICINE PRACTICE

Western herbal practitioners can be accused of creating a myth of herbal medicine as a pure practice. In reality, globally, herbs have always been used alongside any other substances that might achieve therapeutic benefits. Even in contemporary Western herbal medicine, nutritional treatment is seen as an integral part of herbal therapy.

Today in some parts of Europe, most notably France and Germany, a significant number of conventional medical doctors continue to incorporate the prescribing of herbal medicines (as distinct from conventional drugs developed from plants) into their practice. A distinct group of 'Western' herbal practitioners is lacking in many Western countries but is growing in the UK, North America (despite the fact that it is technically illegal for herbalists to practice in the majority of states in the USA) and Australia. The survival, and indeed the growth, of herbal medicine as a discrete discipline in these countries might then be seen as a curiosity, if not an anomaly. It is none the less a testament to the tenacity of herbal practitioners, and to continuing demand from patients.

The fact that Western herbal medicine remains as a viable practice today owes much to the influence of two botanical medicine movements in the USA. These approaches were developed by licensed conventional physicians: namely Eclecticism, developed in the 1820s and operating a school until 1939 (Worthen 2003), and Physiomedicalism, following it in the 1840s. These movements influenced the practice of herbal medicine in the UK, so that when the National Association of Medical Herbalists (later renamed as an Institute rather than an Association) was founded in 1864 it was essentially a Physiomedicalist organization.

This Physiomedicalist approach drew on traditional understanding of herbal medicines (both European and Native American), but also utilized the insights provided by the discovery of the autonomic nervous system to inform the approach to herbal actions and applications (Priest & Priest 1983). In this way, the approach can be seen as modern and even cutting edge. One interpretation of Western herbal medicine's trajectory from this point is that it has continued to develop, working with both traditional knowledge and with that gained from new scientific discoveries. Certainly this is the claim of the approach known as phytotherapy, a term associated with a modern rational approach to herbal medicine.

PROTECTION OF 'TRADITIONAL KNOWLEDGE'

A competing theory, held by some practitioners, is to position herbal medicine as continuing to protect and uphold 'traditional knowledge' against the malign influence of Western scientific thinking. This view of what is meant by 'traditional knowledge' seems to suggest that the notion of 'tradition' is to some extent synonymous with the notion of 'conservation', being guarded and re-enacted in order to be kept alive. In this sense, the practice of medicine becomes a thing deficient in meaning and potency, perhaps like mummers' plays and morris dancing, where the form is retained but the original significance is not fully clear.

There is certainly an important line of thought here, of course, which is significant when looking at indigenous medical practices and their vulnerability to external influence. But is this a legitimate way of regarding the herbal tradition in the UK? The author prefers the view that the Western herbal tradition is dynamic and developing, able to incorporate new data and insights and to respond to changing cultures and changing needs. In this light, herbal medicine can be understood as a modern, living, flexible modality that may be able to continue to be a relevant force in healthcare. Western herbal medicine has only survived to this juncture by virtue of its ability to adapt and innovate.

THE 'MYTH' OF HOLISM

CAM practitioners generally claim to practice holistic medicine, which is often presented as a primary, defining, area of difference with conventional medicine. The word 'holism' was first used by the South African statesman and historian Jan Smuts in 1926 in his book *Holism and evolution*. The concept was developed through work and discussions within Western scientific forums, including conventional medicine. It was eventually appropriated by the CAM movement, which has tended to present the concept simplistically and with little evidence of understanding the origins and issues surrounding the idea (Kaptchuk 2001).

Holism is generally identified with CAM and presented as the contrast to reductionism, which is the practice associated with conventional medicine by CAM authorities. Often, there is little recognition that CAM modalities may be practised in a reductionist manner, and that conventional medicine may be practised holistically. CAM can stand accused of hijacking the scientific knowledge of holism and of appropriating any knowledge arising out of conventional science (such as the understanding of psychoneuroimmunology) when this suits its purposes, often in an unsophisticated manner. If conventional medicine is to be chastised for its reductionism, then CAM might be similarly challenged for an inherent oversimplification. Patrick Pietroni, a conventionally trained medical doctor and one of the leading contemporary proponents of holism, has expressed the view that:

"It is unfortunate that the term holistic medicine has become almost synonymous with alternative medicine and it is important to distinguish between these two epithets."

He goes on to observe that:

"The appeal that many 'alternative therapies' have ... is often based on a misunderstanding of the richness and complexity that underpin the practice of holistic medicine, and has more to do with the search for simple and magical solutions."

(Pietroni 1990)

Mike Webbern, like Pietroni a past Director of the British Holistic Medical Association, has stated that:

"The world of complementary medicine is one which has sat uncomfortably ... on the shoulders of the British Holistic Medical Association which recognises that complementary medicine is not necessarily a part of holism."

(Webbern 1996)

Whilst herbal practitioners, along with other CAM practitioners, may legitimately lay claim to practising holistically and criticize some sectors and practitioners within conventional medicine for failing to do so, they are not justified in appropriating the term. The concept must be shared, not (as we might say) stolen.

THE MYTH OF CAM

In the light of the above, we might refer to the myth of holism in CAM. This leads us to consider the idea of the myth of CAM itself. CAM is generally regarded as a group of contingent practices sharing common aims and principles, but is this really the case? Does the idea of CAM as a homogeneous entity actually hold water? An excellent review of CAM by Kelner et al (2000) concludes that:

"What is important is to recognize that CAM is a complex and constantly changing social phenomenon which defies any arbitrary definition or classification."

None the less, CAM is usually defined by its difference to conventional medicine, but not by the differences within the CAM modalities themselves, which may be very large. Fundamentally, herbal medicine, as a pharmacologically based type of medicine, can be seen as having more in common with conventional medicine (at least in terms of shared understanding of the mechanism of medicines) than with the 'non-material' basis of homoeopathy. Kelner et al (2000) have pointed out that CAM can be defined on its shared beliefs about how the body works, and what constitutes health and disease.

Beliefs provide the foundations of knowledge and there are certainly commonalities across CAM modalities. Most share a belief that the body has self-regulating and self-healing powers, that disease is caused by more than physical factors, and that the spirit–mind–body connection is real and important. However, are these not beliefs that many, if not most, modern conventional medical practitioners also share? Is it not generally the case that the conventional medical research field is the one providing evidence to support these CAM beliefs, for example via studies into the placebo effect and the phenomenon of psychoneuroimmunology?

The difference lies in how practitioners act on these beliefs and how they interpret the responses they get. The practice of acting on and acting out beliefs is, of course, situated in and influenced by constraints such as time, finance and the context of employment. This latter may be more inflexible and restrictive in the public medicine sector (where most conventional medicine is delivered in the UK) than in the private sector (where most CAM is delivered). Such constraints influence practitioners' ability to apply their knowledge, and are influenced by political as well as personal factors. CAM has yet to deal with the challenge that is presented when its medicine has to work with, and within, the infrastructure of mainstream healthcare delivery.

WHICH KNOWLEDGE?

The above sections have suggested that there are varying viewpoints as to what constitutes herbal knowledge. We might though consider which types of knowledge are necessary to suit the agenda of herbal practitioners and the needs of their patients. Clinical research into herbs does not necessarily benefit the herbal profession, since such research, in its conception, execution and presentation, rarely involves herbal practitioners as such. Most of this research is conducted by conventional medical researchers and practitioners, which raises the question – why aren't the fruits of such research then directly incorporated into conventional medical practice? Herbs are after all, as we have discussed previously, pharmacological entities like conventional drugs, and indeed many drugs are already derived from plants. In Germany, this transference of herbal research into conventional medical practice does commonly occur and it may eventually do so in the UK more widely. Werner Busse, as Head of Regulatory and Scientific Affairs at Schwabe Pharmaceuticals, has presented the view that:

"phytomedicines represent part of conventional medicine and as such deserve acceptance as drugs."

(Blumenthal 1997)

Although research into herbal medicines increases the knowledge about the therapeutic uses of plants, it does not necessarily make a case for the practice of herbal medicine as a discrete discipline. In order to enable the development of the profession, herbal practitioners must present data supporting the particular advantages that pertain to the prescribing of herbs by herbal practitioners, rather than others, including the ways in which Western (and other) herbal perspectives can be considered special and desirable (Conway 1998). If herbal medicine is to become a major strand of mainstream medicine in the UK and elsewhere (though of course this goal is not necessarily subscribed to by all herbal practitioners), it will need to achieve several targets.

Herbalists will certainly need to achieve a satisfactory regulatory status, and movement towards this milestone is well under way. For widespread acceptance, it is likely too that herbal medicine research will need to establish the safety, efficacy and economy of treatments according to the criteria set out by the National Institute of Clinical Evidence and other regulatory bodies. Although the clinical evidence base for some herbal medicines is mounting, there is still a great deal of work to be done in this area. Additionally, the particular benefits of herbal medicine prescribed within the context of consultations with herbal practitioners will need to be identified and justified.

In developing a case for the particular approach(es) of herbal medicine, its practitioners will need to consider first principles and map out the philosophical ground upon which the herbal view is constructed. In doing so, it will be necessary to challenge the bias that:

"Medicine never really got anywhere until it threw metaphysics overboard, show me a medical man who still toys with it and I will show you a quack. He may be an ethical quack, but he is still a quack."

(Mencken 1951, quoted in Sherrin 1995)

Unless we can provide a coherent case for our approach – including a convincing philosophical case (see for instance Barker 1991) – then, despite the ethical credibility that statutory self-regulation might confer upon us, herbal practitioners will continue to be seen by some as illegitimate physicians. It is to be hoped that the positive view of Valussi (2001), speaking of research specifically in relation to herbal medicine, is justified when he maintains that:

"The developments in (the) philosophy of science ... have revealed the linguistic, pragmatist and holistic nature of scientific knowledge. It would be impossible nowadays to think of an argumentation ... outside an epistemic framework involving some metaphysical assumptions."

ROUTES TO KNOWLEDGE

Space does not permit a thorough examination of the various ways in which an appropriate evidence base for herbal medicine might best be established. None the less, this section attempts to touch on a few key points about the ways in which beliefs about herbal medicine may achieve the status of knowledge. Knowledge that is seen as trustworthy and meaningful, as well as that which is considered dubious, affects the credibility, status and demand for herbal medicine.

Meaning and mechanism

Harrington (1999), in discussing the problems inherent in a multidisciplinary approach to understanding the placebo effect, makes a statement that is equally applicable to the difficulties that arise in trying to integrate the varying approaches to understanding herbal medicine when she says that:

"The tensions are especially great when one attempts to move between the divide that separates the explanatory strategies of the so-called cultural or hermeneutic sciences (roughly concerned with 'meaning') and the so-called natural sciences (roughly committed to explanations in terms of 'mechanism')."

These divides might also be expressed as empirical versus rational knowledge or as:

"the ongoing and contemporary tensions between two traditions of medical practice identified with the mythical characters Asclepius and Hygeia."
(Dixon & Sweeney 2000)

It is possible, however, to appreciate and utilize the relevance and benefits of each perspective in appropriate circumstances and contexts, rather than committing exclusively to one particular line.

Research strategies and models

The ability of conventional research methodologies to assess adequately and to inform the complexities involved in CAM practice has been frequently questioned by those in the CAM fraternity. Kane (2004), in revisiting arguments addressed above, suggests that this is:

"in part based on the claim that complementary medicine emerges from a holistic philosophy and therefore is not amenable to the scrutiny of the scientific method, which is rooted in a reductionist philosophy."

Certainly, an informed approach to exploring any medical intervention needs to be carefully and sensitively designed and appropriate research strategies have to be used. Glik (2000) has suggested that CAM research models should 'include a broad range of societal factors such as the therapeutic context and the cultural values of patients'. It has been maintained that research methodologies are not sufficiently flexible to assess all the complexities of the herbal treatment approach. Specifically, it is suggested that they do not (or cannot) allow for recognition of the individual variations in treatment and case management and, further, that they do not recognize the influence of the practitioner and the impacts of the therapeutic relationship. The emerging body of reflections and research dealing with the phenomenon of the placebo effect (and the stimulation of the self-healing response) may help to enhance the subtlety and scope of research in these regards (Peters 2001).

The perspectives offered by the 'new science' developing in the fields of quantum mechanics, complexity and chaos theory, and cosmology may well come to inform a more sensitive approach to considering the therapeutic encounter, in its broadest sense and in its details. Developments here can also be seen as providing a bridge between science and mysticism that is of particular relevance to the varied sensibilities and predilections of CAM practitioners. Gleick (1998) further amplifies themes already discussed when he observes that:

"Believers in chaos ... feel that they are turning back a trend in science toward reductionism ... they believe they are looking for the whole."

There are some signs that a specific research perspective for Western herbal medicine is already developing. The EXTRACT database (www.phytotherapy.info), which is currently under construction, shows promise for embodying a credible tailored research resource for herbal medicine. It has reinterpreted the 'level of evidence' criteria of the US Agency for Health Care Policy and Research 1992 from a herbal medicine perspective, and has incorporated into this a rational methodology for grading the traditional (ethnobotanical) records of botanical medicine use.

Evidence-based medicine

Evidence-based medicine (EBM) is the dominant contemporary approach to establishing and legitimizing knowledge in conventional medicine. Its methodology is also being used in herbal medicine (see for instance Rotblatt & Ziment 2002). The originators of the concept have argued that it is a sensitive, and broadly inclusive, approach providing a definition of EBM as 'the integration of best research evidence with clinical expertise and patient values' (Sackett et al 2000). Some have praised it for:

"Its tidy intellectual logic, and apparently simple case, challenging doctors ... to review again the core meaning of medicine. EBM may prove to have been the point when the pendulum of thought started to swing back again from the impersonal aspects of general practice towards the personal."

(Pereira Gray 2000)

Others have taken an opposing view:

"there is no absolute universal notion of science, either in philosophical or historical terms, which should afford a position of unassailable centrality in clinical practice. We accept that the practice and understanding of medicine demands in part a rational appreciation and cognitive evaluation

of information. But it goes beyond that to involve inextricably the self, both the practitioner's self and the patient's self. We argue that the clarity (of EBM) so appealing to politicians is illusory and disingenuous, based on an inadequate explanatory model that is predicated on linear thinking, now recognised to be inappropriate for examining the complexities and constantly evolving nature of the human condition."

(Dixon & Sweeney 2000)

THE APPLICATIONS OF KNOWLEDGE

Individual and group ideology, desires and aspirations provide motives that shape the ends towards which knowledge is employed. The claim of government, and its regulatory apparatus, is that the primary driver underlying the regulation of medical practices is the need to protect the public. To this end, knowledge about what constitutes a safe practitioner and safe practice, and about how such knowledge can be certified and maintained, is paramount. Practitioners tend naturally to take a more practitioner-centric view and may mistrust the ability of a regulatory body to appreciate the complexities of their ethos and work. This may result in a resistance to regulation, based on a view that the regulator will seek to restrict and dictate practice from an ill-informed single-issue perspective. Certainly, public and political pressures will be brought to bear on professions through the regulatory mechanism and these can have major repercussions even for those professions with a long history of statutory regulation. Witness, for example, the upheavals within conventional medicine over recent times in response to a range of serious developments that raise large regulatory questions, such as the Bristol Royal Infirmary children's heart operation scandal, the Alder Hey Children's Hospital organ scandal, and the case of GP Harold Shipman.

When knowledge is not shared, and its premises and applications are disputed, it is hard to find common ground upon which to work collaboratively. Some herbal practitioners align themselves with an alternative worldview such as is manifested in the Green and antiglobalization movements, and rooted in strongly held spiritual or religious convictions. There is a long history of Christian thought influencing Western herbal practice (Kloss 1999). Today, the various emergent (or resurgent) beliefs gathered together under the 'new age' banner exert a profound influence in herbal medicine and other areas of CAM (Hoffmann 1988). Such worldviews are often profoundly sceptical of the dominant Western political systems, their ethos and motives. Seen from such angles, the regulation of herbal practice may be perceived as a phenomenon to be resisted. It is taken as representing the power of the state, operating from a separate and disputed knowledge base, threatening and potentially perverting the identity and meaning of herbal medicine. In any case, is unlikely to have the best interests of herbalism at heart. There may also be a concern that the government, and therefore its regulatory mechanisms, is influenced by powerful players such as the pharmaceutical companies. These may seek to affect herbal practice to suit their own interests.

Whilst it is certainly the case that what is medical is also political, the debate within herbal medicine seems, sometimes, to be characterized by fundamentalism and a lack of sophistication. It appears to be largely based on a deep mistrust of authority and coloured by conspiracy theories. Allied with this is a lack of willingness to engage with the issues formally, preferring instead to remain apart from the apparatus of the state.

It can be contended that this approach has served herbal medicine well in the past (Chapter 9), taking the view that scepticism has aided the survival of herbal medicine. It is therefore understandable that an attachment to such an approach has developed in some cases. We may now, though, be approaching a point where developments in Western scientific thought, medicine and politics are providing an opportunity for herbal medicine to move from the periphery towards the centre, potentially returning to its historical position as a significant strand of mainstream medicine. Herbal medicine has survived, and is now beginning to thrive, in spite of its enforced outsider status. Herbalists have been outsiders by dint of necessity perhaps; but now that the potential exists for significant movement of the profession, a determination to remain in this familiar and comfortable space begins to look less like a credible position, and more like outlaw chic. Are we, as Western herbal practitioners, attached to seeing ourselves as rebels and outsiders, and seduced by the glamour of this? The author has at times despaired of the wilful cultivation of a countercultural stance by some herbalists that would seem to have Patti Smith's rebel shout as its anthem: 'Outside of society, that's where I wanna be' (Smith & Kaye 1978).

It is possible to make a case to support the idea of a strain of noble non-conformism in herbal medicine, but this can become ignoble if the habit is persisted in, against all reason and against the interests of patients and the future of the profession. The claim that modern Western herbal medicine in the UK should be considered as inherently non-conformist is, however, a dubious one. In the 1970s, meetings of the National Institute of Medical Herbalists (the oldest, founded in 1864, and largest of the Western herbal professional associations) were essentially formal black-tie affairs to which local dignitaries were invited (Mills, personal communication, 2003). The Institute was then a conservative medical body focused on upholding the standards of its long tradition of good professional standing in the communities of Britain. Inglis (1964) states that the Institute was founded to: 'improve standards, in order to prove herbalism a reputable alternative to orthodoxy'.

CONCLUSION

The current state of the Western herbal profession in the UK is one of conflicting dynamics, as is perhaps inevitable in a (re)emerging discipline on the cusp of major regulatory developments. Such developments offer huge potential benefits but also challenge varying, but dearly held, beliefs that form differing aspects of the present broad knowledge of herbal medicine. The profession seems both ancient and young at this time, displaying both a well-constructed positive impetus towards enhancing its status and potential, whilst also exhibiting signs of immaturity and a lack of self-confidence and direction. Certainly some of the continuing professional development seminars offered by the profession over the last few years have shown ample evidence of Pietroni's (1990) 'search for simple and magical solutions'.

The profession craves acceptance and approval, on the one hand, whilst demanding acknowledgement of its difference and divergence, on the other. The rapid growth in BSc courses in herbal medicine in the UK (from none in 1994 to seven in 2004) will produce a large influx of new practitioners who will change the landscape of the profession over the coming few years. This prospect can stimulate fear in established practitioners used to a different order of things, and to a lack of competition. Some practitioners may also have been content to practice 'under the radar' and fear the repercussions that might accompany living life in the gradually brightening spotlight. Fear of losing control, and of new impositions, can lead to a defensive and nay-saying reaction. Such are the insecurities and issues of a profession in search of itself, in the process of defining and opening itself and perhaps on the verge of a major breakthrough. Whilst the discussion here suggests that evidence can be gathered to demonstrate a knowledge base capable of taking the weight of regulatory development, there are still lingering questions. Does the current state of the profession really warrant this move now? And are we ready?

References

Barclay J 1909 Southall's organic materia medica. J & A Churchill, London

Barker J 1991 Notes towards a therapeutic model of phytotherapy in Britain. British Journal of Phytotherapy 2(1):25–45

Barker J 2001 The medicinal flora of Britain and Northwestern Europe. Winter Press, West Wickham

Barnes J 2000 Phytotherapy: consumer and pharmacist perspectives. In: Ernst E (ed) Herbal medicine: a concise overview for professionals. Butterworth-Heinemann, Oxford, p 20

Blumenthal M 1997 Testing botanicals. Herbalgram 40:43–46

Conway P 1998 Editorial: towards a new research agenda. European Journal of Herbal Medicine 3(3):2.

Conway P 2001 Book review. British Journal of Phytotherapy, 5(4):223–227

Dixon M, Sweeney K 2000 The human effect in medicine: theory, research and practice. Radcliffe Medical Press, Oxford, p 11

Duke J A 1993 Medicinal plants and the pharmaceutical industry. In: Janick J, Simon, J E (eds) New crops. Wiley, New York, p 664–669

Farnsworth N R, Akerele O, Bingel A S et al 1985 Medicinal plants in therapy. Bulletin of the World Health Organization 63(6):965–981

Fetrow C W, Avila J R 2001 Professional's handbook of complementary and alternative medicines. Lippincott Williams & Wilkins, Philadelphia

General Medical Council 1948 The British pharmacopoeia. Constable, London

Gleick J 1998 Chaos. Vintage, London, p 5

Glik D C 2000 Incorporating symbolic, experiential and social realities into effectiveness research on CAM. In: Kelner M, Wellman B, Pescosolido B et al (eds)

Complementary and alternative medicine: challenge and change. Harwood
Academic, Amsterdam, p 15

Harrington A 1999 Introduction. In: Harrington A (ed) The placebo effect. Harvard
University Press, Cambridge MA, pp 7–8

Herbal Medicine Regulatory Working Group 2003 Recommendations on the
regulation of herbal practitioners in the UK. Prince of Wales's Foundation for
Integrated Health, London

Hindes G 1940 Materia medica and pharmacology for nurses. Faber & Faber, London

Hoffmann D 1988 The holistic herbal. Element Books, Shaftesbury, Dorset

Inglis B 1964 Fringe medicine. Faber & Faber, London, p 69

Kane M 2004 Research made easy in complementary and alternative medicine.
Churchill Livingstone, London, pp 3–4

Kaptchuk T J 2001 History of vitalism In: Micozzi M S (ed) Fundamentals of
complementary and alternative medicine. Churchill Livingstone, London, pp 51–52

Kelner M, Wellman B, Pescosolido B et al 2000 Complementary and alternative
medicine: challenge and change. Harwood Academic, Amsterdam, p 6

Kloss J 1999, first published 1939 Back to Eden. Back to Eden Books, Loma Linda

Newall C A, Anderson L A, Phillipson J D 1996 Herbal medicines: a guide for healthcare professionals. Pharmaceutical Press, London

Pereira Gray D 2000 Introduction. In: Dixon M, Sweeney K (eds) The human effect in
medicine: theory, research and practice. Radcliffe Medical Press, Oxford, p 11

Peters D (ed) 2001 Understanding the placebo effect in complementary medicine:
theory, practice and research. Churchill Livingstone, London

Pietroni P 1990 The greening of medicine. Gollancz, London, pp 25–26

Priest A W, Priest L R 1983 Herbal medication. Fowler, London

Rotblatt M, Ziment I 2002 Evidence-based herbal medicine. Hanley & Belfus, Philadelphia

Sackett D L, Strauss S E, Richardson W S et al 2000 Evidence-based medicine.
Churchill Livingstone, London, p 1

Sherrin N 1995 Oxford dictionary of humorous quotations. Oxford University Press,
Oxford

Smith P, Kaye L 1978 Rock n roll nigger (album track), Easter. Arista Records

Smuts J C 1926 Holism and evolution. Macmillan, London

Thomas K J, Nicholl J P, Coleman P 2001 Use and expenditure on complementary
medicine in England: a population based survey. Complementary Therapies in
Medicine 9(2):11

Valussi M 2001 Biomedical research methods and herbalism: a critique. European
Journal of Herbal Medicine, special issue, pp 25–32

Webbern M 1996 Organizations: the British Holistic Medical Association.
Complementary Therapies in Medicine 4(1):67–68

World Health Organization 2003 Traditional medicine. World Health Organization Fact
Sheet 134. WHO, Geneva

Worthen D B 2003 Fibber McGee's Closet or Tumbling Treasures, Canadian Journal of
Herbalism 24(3):8–11,28

Index

199

Printed and bound by CPI Group (UK) Ltd, Croydon, CR0 4YY

03/10/2024

01040472-0003